400 CALORIE FIX™

DINING GUIDE

Eat Out and Lose Weight with One Simple Rule!

LIZ VACCARIELLO, coauthor of *Flat Belly Diet*®*!*,
with Mindy Hermann, RD, and the editors of **Prevention**®

RODALE

Prevention is a registered trademark of Rodale Inc.
400 Calorie Fix is a trademark of Rodale Inc.

Printed in the United States of America
Rodale Inc. makes every effort to use acid-free ♾, recycled paper ♻.

Photographs: plate images and pages iv–1 © Ted Morrison; pages 8–9 © Vladimir Godnik/gettyimages; pages 14–15 © Fuse/gettyimages; pages 96–97 © Burke/Triolo Productions/gettyimages; pages 166–167 © klaus tiedge/gettyimages.

Book design by Carol Angstadt

Library of Congress Cataloging-in-Publication Data

Vaccariello, Liz.
    400 calorie fix dining guide : eat out and lose weight with one simple rule! / Liz Vaccariello ; with Mindy Hermann and the Editors of Prevention.
        p.   cm.
    ISBN-13: 978-1-60961-009-8 (pbk.)
    ISBN-10: 1-60961-009-1 (pbk.)
    1. Reducing diets.   2. Food—Caloric content.   I. Hermann, Mindy G.   II. Prevention (Emmaus, Pa.)
III. Title.   IV. Title: Four hundred calorie fix dining guide.
RM222.2.V247   2010
613.2'5—dc22   2010031285

2   4   6   8   10   9   7   5   3   1   paperback

We inspire and enable people to improve their lives and the world around them
For more of our products visit rodalestore.com or call 800-848-4735

CONTENTS

Chapter 1

THE 400 CALORIE FIX AT A GLANCE 1

Chapter 2

HOW TO USE THIS GUIDE 9

Chapter 3

DINING OUT 15

Chapter 4

GRABBING A QUICK BITE 97

Chapter 5

HAVING A GOOD TIME 167

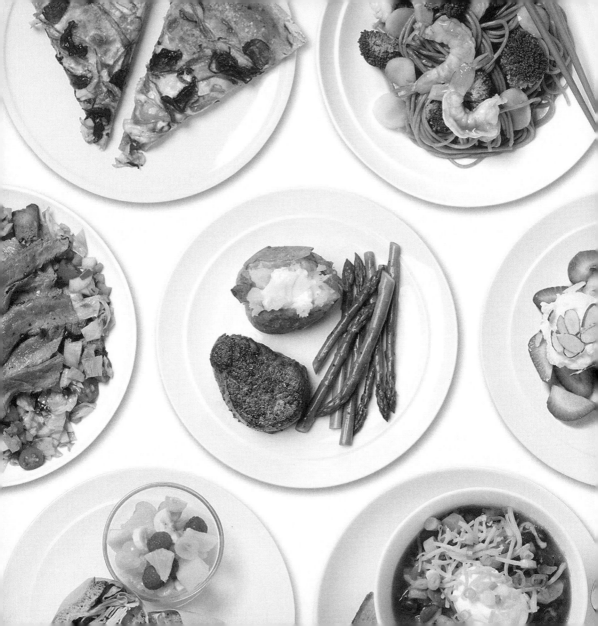

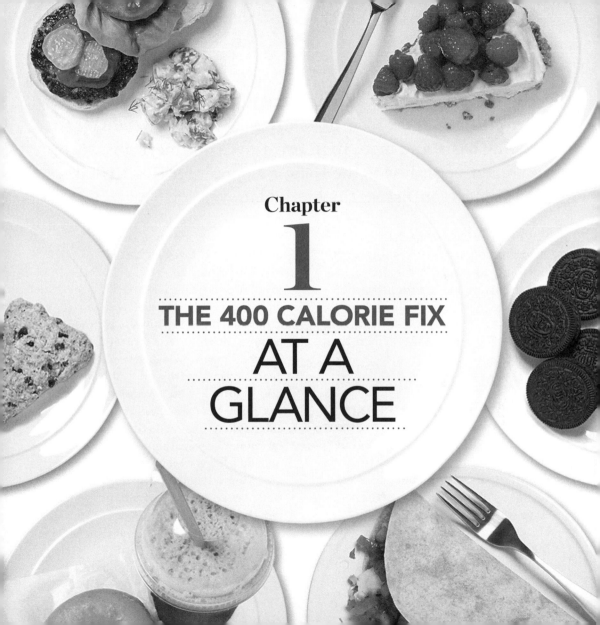

Chapter

1

THE 400 CALORIE FIX

AT A
GLANCE

If you've spent much of your adult life battling extra pounds, you're not alone. Most of us struggle with our weight on an ongoing basis, and more than two-thirds of Americans weigh too much, according to the National Center for Health Statistics, Centers for Disease Control and Prevention.

Why do we have so much trouble shedding pounds and keeping them off? Cutting-edge scientific research has laid the blame on everything from bacteria to hormones to our own genes. But at the root of all of these theories is a very simple answer: We eat more than our bodies need.

WHY CALORIES COUNT

For those of us who are watching our figures, calories have become the enemy. It's certainly true that we eat too many of them. In each of the past 10 years, the average American ate close to 2,700 calories per day, an increase of 500 calories a day since 1970, according to the USDA's Economic Research Service. That daily difference can add up to an extra pound of body fat every week!

Whether they take the form of carbs, protein, or fat, calories clearly matter when you're trying to shed pounds and keep them off. Scientific research keeps coming back to calorie control as the smartest means to losing weight for good. In a landmark study published in 2009, more than 800 overweight adults were assigned to one of four lower-calorie diets: low-fat/high-carb, low-fat/moderate-carb, high-fat/low-carb, and high-fat/very-low-carb. Each diet group lost about the same amount of weight over 2 years, regardless of which diet the group was on.

The problem is, it turns out that counting calories is hard to do—especially when we're eating out. In one study, close to 200 survey respondents who were asked to estimate the calories and fat in nine restaurant entrées were off by more than 100 percent—they thought that a meal with more than 1,300 calories had only 642 calories! Lisa Young, PhD, RD, an adjunct professor of nutrition at New York University, found that most restaurant portions are up to eight times larger than the portions that the government recommends in its Food Guide Pyramid.

That's why I developed the *400 Calorie Fix*, an easy and fun guide that provides you with tools for viewing and choosing food through a healthy calorie lens *without* counting every calorie. As former editor-in-chief of *Prevention* magazine and coauthor of the bestselling *Flat Belly Diet!*, I understand that any eating plan has to fit into your life, not the other way around—which means that you need to be able to take the 400 Calorie Fix out on the town with you. So, once again, I enlisted the help of Mindy Hermann, RD, registered dietitian extraordinaire, to put together a portable *400 Calorie Fix Dining Guide* so you can do just that.

WHY 400 CALORIES IS THE KEY

If you grew up on 1,000-calorie burgers or plates of pasta, 400 calories probably sounds like a starvation diet. But if you've tried any of the meals in our first two books, *400 Calorie Fix* or *400 Calorie Fix Cookbook,* you already know that 400 calories is the perfect per-meal "fix," with enough food and calories to provide the energy you need and keep you satiated until your next meal. If you're new to the 400 Calorie Fix, we promise you'll be pleasantly surprised by how full you can feel on 400 calories. You'll find that 400 calories gives you plenty of room for variety so that you can enjoy different tastes, textures, and nutrients at each meal. And you don't need to give up anything; you can have your cake (and cheese and chocolate and cocktails, too) and still lose weight on the 400 Calorie Fix. In fact, when we asked some of our readers to test the plan for us, they lost an average of 6 pounds in just 2 weeks, with several shedding up to 11 pounds—and they did it eating pizza, steak, and chocolate chip scones!

"How Many Meals Should I Eat?"

Women

WEIGHT GOAL/ ACTIVITY LEVEL	SEDENTARY	SOMEWHAT ACTIVE/ACTIVE	VERY ACTIVE
Lose	3 meals	3–4 meals	4 meals
Maintain	3–4 meals	4 meals	4–5 meals

Men

WEIGHT GOAL/ ACTIVITY LEVEL	SEDENTARY	SOMEWHAT ACTIVE/ACTIVE	VERY ACTIVE
Lose	3–4 meals	4 meals	4–5 meals
Maintain	4 meals	4–5 meals	5+ meals

SEDENTARY: You sit most of the day and drive everywhere, and you log plenty of hours of screen time each day.

SOMEWHAT ACTIVE: You get about 30 minutes of physical activity daily. Nothing too strenuous, generally the equivalent of walking about 1½ to 3 miles daily, or 3,000 to 6,000 steps on a pedometer.

ACTIVE: You like to move around and clock 30 to 60 minutes of daily physical activity by hitting the gym, climbing stairs at the office, and parking farther away at the market along with moderate exercise, the equivalent of walking more than 3 miles per day, or more than 6,000 steps on a pedometer.

VERY ACTIVE: You're more than a weekend warrior; you thrive on high-intensity sports and rigorous activities that total more than 60 minutes per day.

The 400-calorie meal also fits neatly into your daily calorie needs. A woman who is of average size and average activity level and wants to maintain her weight needs about 1,600 calories per day; that's four 400-calorie meals a day. The average man needs about 2,000 calories a day, or five 400-calorie meals. To lose weight, cut out one meal. (See the *400 Calorie Fix* for specifics on the 2 Week Quick Slim program for weight loss.)

Consult the chart above to determine the number of 400-calorie meals you should eat per day, and hence, your daily calorie count. (To find out more about your daily calorie needs, visit www.prevention.com/healthtracker.)

THE 400 CALORIE FIX TOOLBOX

In *400 Calorie Fix,* we introduced five tools to help you find 400-calorie meals anywhere you go, whether you're out celebrating with friends or running errands. Three of these tools are featured in this book. You can find information on the other two tools, the 2 Week Quick Slim (a set menu providing 1,200 calories a day) and 400 Calorie Menus (daily meal plans based on different eating styles), in *400 Calorie Fix.*

The three tools we highlight in this book are particularly useful for our busy lifestyle. It's easy to control calories if you have all the time in the world to cook healthy and hearty meals for yourself and your family, but we know real life doesn't work that way. So we designed these tools for you to use when you're out and about.

400 Calorie Meals. With more than 150 meals to eat on the go, organized into sections on dining out (Chapter 3), grabbing a quick bite (Chapter 4), and having a good time (Chapter 5), we promise you'll have plenty to eat no matter where you go.

We combed through a wide range of sit-down restaurants, fast-food chains, and fun settings like ball games, boardwalks, and bars to highlight 400-calorie meals that you can enjoy wherever you are. Looking for 400 calories in a Chinese restaurant? Try Shrimp with Candied Walnuts (page 84), with enough calories left to start with a chicken lettuce wrap. Cheering on your favorite team? The Hot Dog meal (page 177) includes a ballpark dog plus beer.

400 Calorie Lens. These simple visual tricks and shortcuts help you gauge how much food really adds up to 400 calories.

Estimating food portions and calories is tough, especially when you're eating out. After all, you can't bring a set of measuring cups into a restaurant! So you'll be using our visual cues (page 12) to estimate restaurant portion sizes. In addition, use them to train your eye at home so that you'll be better equipped on the go.

4 Star Nutrition System. Although it's calories that count for weight loss, nutrition still matters to keep you healthy, happy, and satisfied while you shed the pounds. The 4 Star Nutrition System is a simple way to give you a healthy balance of the four important components in healthy meals—protein, fiber, good fats, and fruits and vegetables—throughout the day.

Meals that meet the criteria for each category are starred accordingly.

★ Protein—meals with at least 20 grams of protein
★ Fiber—meals that have at least 7 grams of fiber
★ Good fats—meals that contain either a major source of monounsaturated fatty acids or at least 2 teaspoons of olive oil per serving
★ Fruits/veggies—meals with at least 1 cup of fruits and vegetables

You will notice that some meals have just one star while others have two, three, even four stars because they qualify in more than one category. And many on-the-go meals have no stars. In fact, restaurants, fast food, and take-out vendors could do a much better job at putting higher nutrition options on their menus. Getting enough fiber and good fats when you're eating on the go is particularly challenging. Do your best to collect each category at least once during the day through a combination of foods on the go and foods eaten at home or work and you'll be on the road to healthy eating.

You're more likely to stick to a diet that fits your lifestyle and helps you make smart food choices wherever you are. The *400 Calorie Fix Dining Guide* does just that by giving you information on foods that are likely to be on the menus of restaurants, fast-food outlets, and fun away-from-home locations. Pair the *400 Calorie Fix Dining Guide* with *400 Calorie Fix* and *400 Calorie Fix Cookbook* for a complete food survival guide.

FIXES

1 Look up calorie info ahead of time on the restaurant Web site. No Web site? Look for one with similar foods.

2 Fill up on raw vegetables before you leave the house.

3 Start your meal with a fruit or veggie appetizer.

4 Share with a friend. Many restaurant meals supply at least twice your 400 calories.

5 Ask about sauce ingredients and order sauces on the side when possible.

6 Dish out your food onto an appetizer-size plate. When plates are bigger, we tend to eat more.

7 Order coffee or tea to end your meal, plus one small dessert for the table.

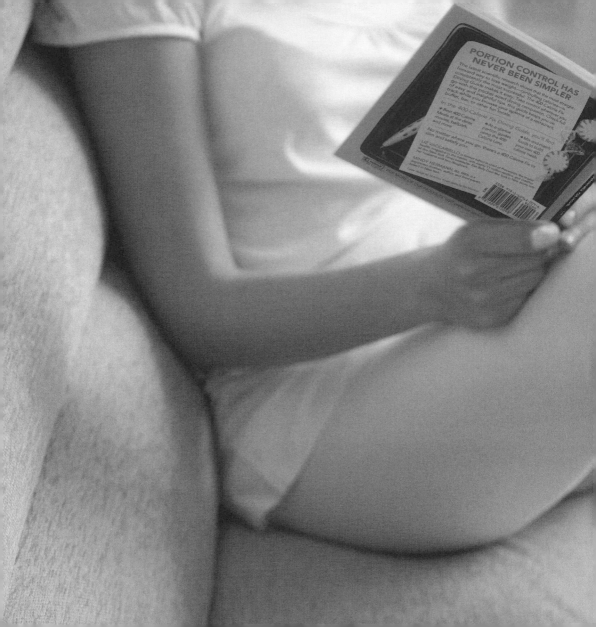

**PORTION CONTROL HAS
NEVER BEEN SIMPLER**

The latest scientific research shows that the most straight-
forward way to lose weight—controlling the calories you
eat—probably the most successful. The 400 calorie fix
Dining Guide makes it even easier. Take the 400 calorie
go-well this pocket-sized companion wherever you go so it's
so easy and helpful tips like drinking your options and to
track while you indulge. Use your options at a restaurant,
buffet, bar, or other fun foods.

In the *400 Calorie Fix Dining Guide*, you'll find:

• Best 400 Calorie   • Wine glasses   • Mix-and-match
  Meals at chain   pairing the 400   foods to total
  restaurants,   Calorie Fix   400
  bakeries, delis,   calorie meals
  and more

No matter where you go, there's a 400 Calorie Fix to
calm and satisfy you.

LIZ VACCARIELLO is editor-in-chief of *Prevention* magazine and the
author of the *New York Times* bestsellers *Flat Belly Diet!* and *400
Calorie Fix.* She lives outside of New York City with her husband and
their two daughters.

MINDY HERMANN, RD, MBA, is a
registered dietitian for family. She has the look to talk about
nutrition, where and often has.

Chapter
2
HOW TO
USE THIS
GUIDE

A s we all know from experience, the most difficult time to stick to a calorie goal is when you're eating away from home. Sometimes it's hard to pass up the cheesy goodness of nachos or the chocolatey indulgence of brownies, even though we know they'll break our calorie budget. And you know what? It's okay to eat a 400-calorie meal of ice cream once in a while.

But sometimes we overdo the calories because we don't know how many are in a dish that someone else prepared. That's where the *400 Calorie Fix Dining Guide* comes in. Our mission is to help you put together 400-calorie meals anywhere—at your favorite restaurant, at parties, even at notoriously unhealthy places like the bar, the movies, and the county fair. So we tailored the 400 Calorie Fix Toolbox to be especially useful when you're eating out.

YOUR 400 CALORIE WORLD

As you'll see, the book is organized into sections that correspond with restaurants or other settings where you may have limited food options. In each section, you'll find a list of foods and dishes commonly found in that place. For example, in the Italian restaurant section, you'll find pepperoni, minestrone soup, pasta Bolognese, chicken Marsala, and tiramisu.

Each dish is listed in three different portions. The *typical portion* estimates the amount that you might be served in the restaurant and often exceeds 400 calories. In most Italian restaurants, for instance, you get a large bowl full of linguine with white clam sauce. The bowl contains about 2 cups of pasta with sauce, which is 1,020 calories. Of course, this calorie count varies from restaurant to restaurant, depending upon both the amount of food they dish up and the ingredients they use in cooking the food, so what we're showing you here are averages based upon information we've researched from several popular restaurant chains.

The *400-calorie portion* is the quantity of food that you could eat if you do choose to devote one entire meal to just one food. Remember we said it was okay to eat a 400-calorie meal of nothing but ice cream occasionally? Well, 1⅛ cups of gelato will fill that bill nicely.

If, however, you're looking to build a more balanced meal, use the *meal portion* to guide you. For example, if you eat just half a piece of meat lasagna at 240 calories, that will give you room to add a cup of soup or a garden side salad plus maybe even a few bites of bread.

Dishes with more than one food, such as a hamburger topped with lettuce and tomato, display each food separated by a "+" sign (i.e., hamburger + lettuce + tomato). These are easiest to customize by ordering more or less of some foods to suit your tastes—and your desired calorie count. As you'll learn, some foods are particularly high in calories, so whenever it's possible to omit them

from your order without sacrificing taste, we suggest (in the meal portions) that you do so. But we won't ask you to pick out all the meat from your spaghetti. When foods are so mixed together that it's impossible to separate them, we'll simply suggest eating a smaller portion of the whole dish.

I know this may seem like a lot of numbers for a guide in which we promised you wouldn't have to count calories. We wanted to give you enough information so that you could mix and match foods to suit your own tastes. But if that feels like too much work for you, try one of our 400 Calorie Meal combos. You'll see those meals in the margins throughout each section.

Each of these meals is marked with stars as part of the 4 Star Nutrition System. Some cuisines are absolutely stellar in their variety of picks that are high in nutrition. For example, Mexican food offers plenty of vegetables, lots of fiber from beans and corn tortillas, and good fats in the form of avocado. Other cuisines fall short. Your goal is to collect at least one of each star every day—if your only on-the-go choices have no

It's a Ball, It's a Hand, It's a Portion!

Ball	Hand	Portion	Examples	
Small marble	tip of the thumb	1 teaspoon	oil, butter, margarine	
Large marble	thumb to the first knuckle	1 tablespoon	chopped nuts, ketchup, mustard, mayonnaise	
2 large marbles	whole thumb	2 tablespoons/ 1 fluid ounce liquid	grated cheese, raisins	
Golf ball	cupped handful	¼ cup	salsa, hummus, guacamole	
Hockey puck	palm of the hand	½ cup/3–4 ounces cooked meat, poultry, fish	burger patty, beef, pork, chicken, turkey, fish	
Tennis ball	open handful	½ cup	pasta, rice, small potato, small roll	
Wiffle ball	very loose cupped handful	1 cup/1–2 ounces chips	cotton candy, popcorn	
Baseball	whole fist	1 cup	soup, lettuce, vegetables, fruit	

stars, you'll need to gather all four stars from your other meals that day.

SEEING 400 CALORIES

Most of the portions in the book are given in volume measurements (teaspoons, tablespoons, and cups). Some foods, such as meat, poultry, and fish, are measured by weight. But since we don't expect you to bring a measuring cup or food scale with you to the restaurant, use the visual cues in the chart on page 12 to help you eyeball the correct portions.

ADDITIONAL FEATURES

400 Calorie Tips and Fixes. Each food section includes tips and fixes that are specific to that cuisine or setting. You'll learn which foods add extra nutrition, how to select foods within a 400-calorie framework, and how to mix and match foods to suit your tastes.

Find the Fat, Spot the Sugar. Picking foods lower in fat and sugar allows you to have bigger portions

without too many extra calories. Look for the Find the Fat and Spot the Sugar feature throughout the book for guidance on making the best food choices.

Bite by Bite. If you're a nibbler, you'll benefit from information on just how many calories are in a bite of favorite foods like desserts and fast-food items.

THE 1-2-3-400
CALORIE TRICK

You can use the 1-2-3-400 Calorie Trick to get close to 400 calories at settings where you're eating small amounts of lots of different foods.

- Mentally divide your plate into six sections.
- Fill **1** section with proteins like meat, chicken, and fish.
- Fill **2** sections with grain foods such as rice, pasta, and bread.
- Fill **3** sections with vegetables and fruit.

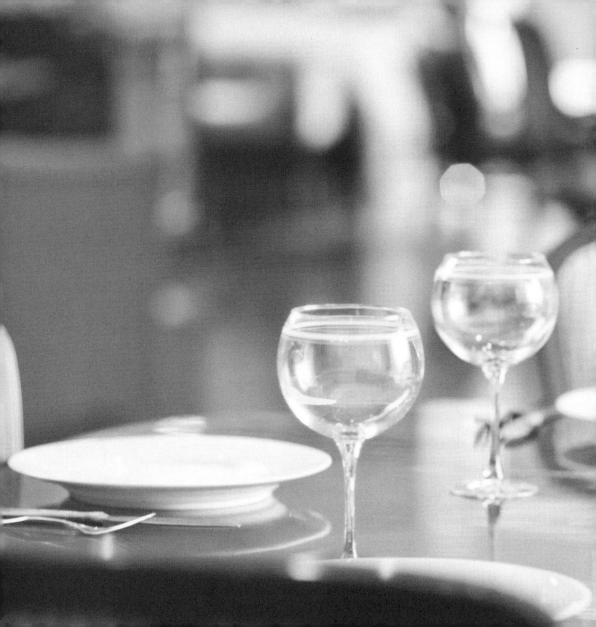

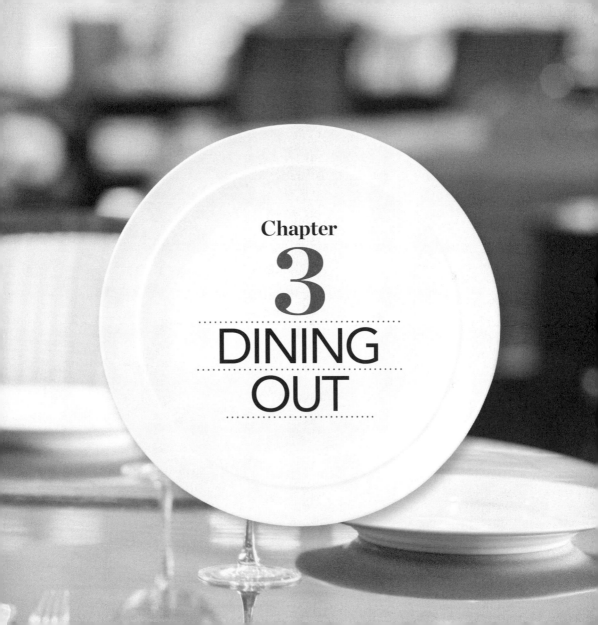

Chapter

3

DINING OUT

AMERICAN

American fare, including the classics and more

Sharpen your portion-control skills before heading to an American restaurant. Servings of appetizers, main dishes, sides, and desserts tend to be oversized, with enough food and calories to serve four or more people. The appetizer menu in particular is filled with choices that are extremely high in calories; it's best to take just a bite or to say no altogether. Keep your order simple—the more elaborate the dish, the more likely it is to be packed with calories.

TYPICAL PORTION	400-CALORIE PORTION	MEAL PORTION

APPETIZERS

SHRIMP COCKTAIL

3 shrimp + ¼ cup cocktail sauce	12 shrimp + 1 cup cocktail sauce	3 shrimp + ¼ cup cocktail sauce
90 calories	*360 calories*	*90 calories*

FRIED CALAMARI

1½ cups	1½ cups	½ cup
400 calories	*400 calories*	*130 calories*

STUFFED POTATO SKINS

4 skins	6 skins	2 skins
280 calories	*420 calories*	*140 calories*

JUMBO STUFFED MUSHROOMS

3 mushrooms	2½ mushrooms	1 mushroom
500 calories	*420 calories*	*170 calories*

SPINACH ARTICHOKE DIP AND LAVOSH CRACKERS

2 cups dip + 25 pieces lavosh	½ cup dip + 7 pieces lavosh	¼ cup dip + 3 pieces lavosh
1,360 calories	*390 calories*	*170 calories*

BUFFALO CHICKEN WINGS

8 wings + ¼ cup blue cheese dressing	5 wings + 2 Tbsp blue cheese dressing	2 wings + 1 Tbsp blue cheese dressing
680 calories	*425 calories*	*170 calories*

Spinach Dip and Salad

¼ cup spinach artichoke dip + 3 pieces lavosh crackers
170

+

Chopped side salad (2 cups + 1 tsp olive oil + vinegar to taste)
230

=

400
calories
★ *fruits/veggies*

Cheeseburger Slider

1 cheeseburger slider
210

.... + ...

Large spinach salad
(2 cups spinach
+ 1 egg + 1 Tbsp blue
cheese + 1 tsp olive oil
+ vinegar to taste)
170

.... = ...

380

calories

★ *fruits/veggies*

Skip the noodles in chicken noodle soup to get the satiating benefits of soup while cutting out about half the calories.

	TYPICAL PORTION	400-CALORIE PORTION	MEAL PORTION
HUMMUS WITH MEDIUM (6½") PITA			
	1 cup hummus + 2 pitas	½ cup hummus + 1 pita	¼ cup hummus + ½ pita
	750 calories	*380 calories*	*190 calories*
MOZZARELLA STICKS			
	10 sticks + ½ cup marinara sauce	4 sticks + 6 Tbsp marinara sauce	2 sticks + 3 Tbsp marinara sauce
	870 calories	*390 calories*	*195 calories*
CHEESEBURGER SLIDERS			
	6 sliders	2 sliders	1 slider
	1,260 calories	*420 calories*	*210 calories*

SOUPS

	TYPICAL PORTION	400-CALORIE PORTION	MEAL PORTION
CHICKEN NOODLE SOUP			
	1 bowl (1½ cups)	4 cups	1 bowl (1½ cups)
	160 calories	*400 calories*	*160 calories*
BAKED POTATO SOUP			
	1 bowl (1½ cups)	1 bowl (1½ cups)	½ bowl (¾ cup)
	370 calories	*370 calories*	*185 calories*

TYPICAL PORTION	400-CALORIE PORTION	MEAL PORTION
FRENCH ONION SOUP		
1 bowl (1½ cups)	2 cups	1 bowl (1½ cups)
280 calories	*370 calories*	*280 calories*
NEW ENGLAND CLAM CHOWDER		
1 bowl (1½ cups)	1⅓ cups	1 cup
450 calories	*400 calories*	*300 calories*

SALADS

SMALL FIELD GREENS SALAD		
1 cup field greens + 1 Tbsp each dried cranberries, pecans + 1 Tbsp vinaigrette	3 salads	1 cup field greens + 1 Tbsp each dried cranberries, pecans + 1 Tbsp balsamic vinegar
125 calories	*375 calories*	*95 calories*
LARGE SALAD		
2 cups lettuce + 8 tomato wedges + 4 Tbsp ranch dressing	2½ cups lettuce + 10 tomato wedges + 5 Tbsp ranch dressing	2 cups lettuce + 4 tomato wedges + 2 tsp olive oil + vinegar to taste
340 calories	*425 calories*	*130 calories*

Soup and Salad

1 bowl
French onion soup
280

+

Small field greens salad
(1 cup field greens
+ 1 Tbsp each
dried cranberries,
pecans + 1 Tbsp
balsamic vinegar)
95

+

1 cup fresh strawberries
50

=

425
calories

★ *good fats*
★ *fruits/veggies*

Chef's Salad

Chef's salad
(4 cups romaine +
4 tomato wedges +
1 oz each turkey, ham,
roast beef + 1 egg +
1 tsp olive oil +
1 Tbsp
balsamic vinegar)
260

·········· + ··········

Medium dinner roll +
2 pats butter
160

========= = =========

420
calories

★ protein
★ fruits/veggies

	TYPICAL PORTION	400-CALORIE PORTION	MEAL PORTION
LARGE SPINACH SALAD			
	2 cups spinach + 1 egg + 2 Tbsp blue cheese + 4 Tbsp blue cheese dressing	2 cups spinach + 1 egg + 2 Tbsp blue cheese + 3 Tbsp blue cheese dressing	2 cups spinach + 1 egg + 1 Tbsp blue cheese + 1 tsp olive oil + vinegar to taste
	445 calories	*375 calories*	*170 calories*
CHOPPED SIDE SALAD with assorted vegetables and Cheddar cheese			
	2 cups + 2 Tbsp ranch dressing	1 salad	2 cups + 1 tsp olive oil + vinegar to taste
	360 calories	*360 calories*	*230 calories*
CHEF'S SALAD			
	4 cups romaine + 4 tomato wedges + 2 oz each turkey, ham, roast beef + 2 sliced eggs + ¼ cup sliced American cheese + 2 Tbsp sliced olives + 4 Tbsp ranch dressing	½ chef's salad	4 cups romaine + 4 tomato wedges + 1 oz each turkey, ham, roast beef + 1 egg + 1 tsp olive oil + 1 Tbsp balsamic vinegar
	850 calories	*425 calories*	*260 calories*

TYPICAL PORTION	400-CALORIE PORTION	MEAL PORTION
ASIAN GRILLED CHICKEN SALAD with greens, fried wonton strips, almond slivers, and chicken strips		
4 cups salad + 4 Tbsp Asian vinaigrette dressing	½ salad + 1 Tbsp Asian vinaigrette dressing	½ salad, no dressing
1,310 calories	*400 calories*	*320 calories*
GRILLED CHICKEN CAESAR		
4 cups romaine + 6 oz chicken + 1 Tbsp croutons + 4 Tbsp Caesar dressing	2 cups romaine + 3 oz chicken + 1 Tbsp croutons + 2 Tbsp Caesar dressing	2 cups romaine + 3 oz chicken + 1 Tbsp croutons + 2 Tbsp Caesar dressing
820 calories	*410 calories*	*410 calories*

Asian Grilled Chicken Salad

½ Asian grilled chicken salad, without dressing
320

+

Medium dinner roll
100

=

420
calories

★ *protein*
★ *fruits/veggies*

Regular Caesar dressing is one of the highest-calorie dressings because it is made mostly from oil.

Turkey Dinner

1 bowl
chicken noodle soup
160
.... + ...
3 oz turkey breast
+ 2 Tbsp gravy
125
.... + ...
½ large
baked potato
140
.... = ...

425
calories
★ *protein*

	TYPICAL PORTION	400-CALORIE PORTION	MEAL PORTION

ENTREÉS

SHRIMP SCAMPI

TYPICAL PORTION	400-CALORIE PORTION	MEAL PORTION
1½ cups	3¾ cups	¾ cup
160 calories	*400 calories*	*80 calories*

GRILLED MAHI MAHI

TYPICAL PORTION	400-CALORIE PORTION	MEAL PORTION
10 oz	13 oz	3 oz
300 calories	*390 calories*	*90 calories*

GRILLED TUNA

TYPICAL PORTION	400-CALORIE PORTION	MEAL PORTION
10 oz	11 oz	3 oz
370 calories	*410 calories*	*110 calories*

SWORDFISH STEAK

TYPICAL PORTION	400-CALORIE PORTION	MEAL PORTION
8 oz	9 oz	3 oz
350 calories	*390 calories*	*130 calories*

GRILLED TILAPIA FILLET

TYPICAL PORTION	400-CALORIE PORTION	MEAL PORTION
10 oz	11 oz	3 oz
370 calories	*410 calories*	*110 calories*

STEAMED LOBSTER

TYPICAL PORTION	400-CALORIE PORTION	MEAL PORTION
Meat from 1 lb lobster + ¼ cup melted butter	Meat from 1 lb lobster + 3 Tbsp melted butter	Meat from 1 lb lobster
520 calories	*410 calories*	*110 calories*

TYPICAL PORTION	400-CALORIE PORTION	MEAL PORTION
ROTISSERIE CHICKEN		
½ breast + 1 leg	½ breast, no skin	1 drumstick, no skin
500 calories	*370 calories*	*110 calories*
PORK TENDERLOIN		
8 oz	10 oz	3 oz
320 calories	*400 calories*	*120 calories*

BE STINGY WITH
SAUCES

High-fat or high-sugar sauces and dressings can add unwanted calories to your meal, so use them sparingly or not at all.

1 Tbsp gravy	10 calories
1 Tbsp shrimp cocktail sauce	15 calories
1 Tbsp marinara sauce	15 calories
1 Tbsp steak sauce	20 calories
1 Tbsp béarnaise sauce	40 calories
1 Tbsp blue cheese dressing	70 calories
1 Tbsp tartar sauce	80 calories
1 Tbsp melted butter	90 calories

Shrimp Scampi

Large salad
(2 cups lettuce
+ 4 tomato wedges
+ 2 tsp olive oil
+ vinegar to taste)
130
+

1½ cups
shrimp scampi
160
+

½ cup pasta
110
=

400
calories
★ *fruits/veggies*

Pot Roast

3 oz pot roast
170
·········· **+** ··········
½ cup roasted new potatoes
100
·········· **+** ··········
½ slice apple pie
150
·········· **=** ··········

420
calories
★ *protein*

TYPICAL PORTION	400-CALORIE PORTION	MEAL PORTION
ROASTED TURKEY BREAST WITH GRAVY		
6 oz + ¼ cup gravy	9 oz + 6 Tbsp gravy	3 oz + 2 Tbsp gravy
245 calories	*375 calories*	*125 calories*
GRILLED CHICKEN BREAST		
6 oz	9 oz	3 oz
280 calories	*420 calories*	*140 calories*
LONDON BROIL		
12 oz	7 oz	3 oz
680 calories	*400 calories*	*170 calories*
POT ROAST		
8 oz	7 oz	3 oz
460 calories	*400 calories*	*170 calories*
PORTERHOUSE STEAK		
12 oz	6⅔ oz	3 oz
720 calories	*400 calories*	*180 calories*
GRILLED SALMON FILLET		
10 oz	6⅔ oz	3 oz
600 calories	*400 calories*	*180 calories*
FILET MIGNON		
8 oz	6⅓ oz	3 oz
500 calories	*400 calories*	*190 calories*

TYPICAL PORTION	400-CALORIE PORTION	MEAL PORTION
PORK CHOP		
8 oz	6 oz	3 oz
530 calories	*400 calories*	*200 calories*
FRIED SHRIMP		
15 shrimp	12 shrimp	6 shrimp
500 calories	*400 calories*	*200 calories*
RIB EYE STEAK		
12 oz	5¾ oz	3 oz
840 calories	*400 calories*	*210 calories*

Filet Mignon

3 shrimp + ¼ cup
cocktail sauce
90
················· + ·················
Small field greens salad
(1 cup field greens +
1 Tbsp each dried
cranberries, pecans +
1 Tbsp vinaigrette)
125
················· + ·················
3 oz filet mignon
190
················· = ·················

405
calories

★ *protein*
★ *good fats*
★ *fruits/veggies*

BUFFET DINING

Calories add up quickly at the buffet table, especially if you enjoy taking at least a taste of almost everything. To keep things under control:

- Fill at least half your plate with veggies.
- Choose dishes that don't have the glossy sheen of added butter or oil.
- Limit grains and starches to a flat serving spoon.
- Limit the total size of your main dish portion to the palm of your hand.

Chili

1 cup chili +
1 Tbsp Cheddar cheese
+ 1 Tbsp sour cream
260
.... **+** ....
2 saltine crackers
25
.... **+** ....
1 bottle light beer
100
.... **=** ....

385

calories

★ *protein*
★ *fiber*

TYPICAL PORTION	400-CALORIE PORTION	MEAL PORTION
CHICKEN FRIED STEAK WITH GRAVY		
8 oz steak + ¼ cup gravy	5 oz steak + 3 Tbsp gravy	3 oz steak + 2 Tbsp gravy
595 calories	*390 calories*	*235 calories*
CHILI with Cheddar cheese and sour cream		
1 bowl chili (2 cups) + 3 Tbsp Cheddar cheese + 2 Tbsp sour cream	¾ bowl chili (1½ cups) + 1 Tbsp Cheddar cheese + 1 Tbsp sour cream	1 cup chili + 1 Tbsp Cheddar cheese + 1 Tbsp sour cream
540 calories	*370 calories*	*260 calories*
SURF AND TURF (rib eye steak and lobster)		
5 oz steak + meat from ½ lobster	5 oz steak + meat from ½ lobster	3 oz steak + meat from ½ lobster
400 calories	*400 calories*	*260 calories*
BABY BACK RIBS		
4 ribs	2¾ ribs	2 ribs
620 calories	*410 calories*	*310 calories*

TYPICAL PORTION	400-CALORIE PORTION	MEAL PORTION

SIDE DISHES

GRILLED ASPARAGUS

5 spears	55 spears	5 spears
35 calories	*385 calories*	*35 calories*

STEAMED GREEN BEANS

1 cup + 1 pat butter	10 cups	1 cup
70 calories	*400 calories*	*40 calories*

STEAMED BROCCOLI

1 cup + 2 Tbsp cheese sauce	8 cups, no sauce	1 cup, no sauce
110 calories	*400 calories*	*50 calories*

GLAZED CARROTS

1 cup	5 cups	1 cup
80 calories	*400 calories*	*80 calories*

MASHED POTATOES

1 cup + 1 pat butter	2 cups + 2 pats butter	½ cup
210 calories	*420 calories*	*90 calories*

SAUTÉED MIXED VEGETABLES

1 cup	4½ cups	1 cup
90 calories	*405 calories*	*90 calories*

Grilled Tuna and Glazed Carrots

3 oz grilled tuna
110

+

1 cup glazed carrots
80

+

⅔ cup brown rice
150

+

1 cup cappuccino made with fat-free milk
40

=

380
calories

★ protein
★ good fats
★ fruits/veggies

Pork and Potatoes

3 oz pork tenderloin
120

.... + ...

½ cup roasted new
potatoes
100

.... + ...

5 spears grilled
asparagus
35

.... + ...

1 chocolate chip cookie
140

.... = ...

395
calories

★ *protein*
★ *fruits/veggies*

TYPICAL PORTION	400-CALORIE PORTION	MEAL PORTION
ROASTED NEW POTATOES		
1 cup	2 cups	½ cup
200 calories	*400 calories*	*100 calories*
MEDIUM DINNER ROLL		
1 roll + 2 pats butter	2½ rolls + 5 pats butter	1 roll
160 calories	*400 calories*	*100 calories*
PASTA		
1 cup	1¾ cups	½ cup
220 calories	*390 calories*	*110 calories*
WHITE RICE		
1 cup	2 cups	⅔ cup
200 calories	*400 calories*	*130 calories*
RICE PILAF		
1 cup	1½ cups	½ cup
280 calories	*420 calories*	*140 calories*
LARGE BAKED POTATO (10½ OZ)		
1 potato + 1 pat butter + 2 Tbsp sour cream	1 potato + 1 pat butter + 2 Tbsp sour cream	½ potato, no butter or sour cream
390 calories	*390 calories*	*140 calories*

TYPICAL PORTION	400-CALORIE PORTION	MEAL PORTION
BROWN RICE		
1 cup *220 calories*	1¾ cups *390 calories*	⅔ cup *150 calories*
LARGE (1 LB) BLOOMING ONION		
1 onion *1,520 calories*	¼ onion *380 calories*	¼ onion *380 calories*

For more fiber to keep you full, choose brown rice over white and new potatoes rather than mashed.

LOOKING FOR
MUFAS?

Monounsaturated fatty acids (or, as I like to call them, MUFAs) are a type of fat that is important to health. Research shows that MUFAs aid weight loss. They also help protect your heart. So seek out MUFAs (and another healthy fat, omega-3 fatty acids) in these foods:

- Avocado
- Dark chocolate
- Fatty fish
- Olives
- Nuts

Roast Chicken

3 oz roast chicken breast
140

·········· **+** ··········

½ cup mashed potatoes
+ 1 pat butter
120

·········· **+** ··········

1 cup sautéed mixed vegetables
90

·········· **+** ··········

1 cup fresh strawberries
50

·········· **=** ··········

400
calories

★ *protein*
★ *fruits/veggies*

TYPICAL PORTION	400-CALORIE PORTION	MEAL PORTION
DESSERTS		
FRESH STRAWBERRIES		
1 cup + 2 Tbsp whipped cream	4 cups + ½ cup whipped cream	1 cup, no whipped cream
100 calories	*400 calories*	*50 calories*
ICE CREAM AND SORBET		
½ cup premium ice cream	2½ cups sorbet	½ cup sorbet
270 calories	*400 calories*	*80 calories*
FRUIT SALAD		
1 cup	4 cups	1 cup
100 calories	*400 calories*	*100 calories*
SMALL (1 OZ) CHOCOLATE CHIP COOKIES		
3 cookies	3 cookies	1 cookie
420 calories	*420 calories*	*140 calories*
9" APPLE PIE (CUT INTO 8 SLICES)		
1 slice + 1 scoop vanilla ice cream (½ cup)	1 slice + 2 Tbsp vanilla ice cream	½ slice
570 calories	*370 calories*	*150 calories*

TYPICAL PORTION	400-CALORIE PORTION	MEAL PORTION
9" KEY LIME PIE (CUT INTO 8 SLICES)		
1 slice	1 slice	½ slice
420 calories	*420 calories*	*210 calories*
9" CHOCOLATE MOUSSE CAKE (CUT INTO 14 SLICES)		
1 slice	1 slice	½ slice
510 calories	*510 calories*	*255 calories*
6" CHEESECAKE (CUT INTO 6 SLICES)		
1 slice	1½ slices	1 slice
260 calories	*390 calories*	*260 calories*

All desserts are high in calories, so pick your favorite and eat just a few bites to satisfy your craving.

Grilled Tilapia

3 oz grilled tilapia
110

················· **+** ·················

½ cup roasted
new potatoes
100

················· **+** ·················

1 cup sautéed
mixed vegetables
90

················· **+** ·················

1 glass wine
120

················· **=** ·················

420
calories

★ *protein*
★ *fruits/veggies*

TYPICAL PORTION	400-CALORIE PORTION	MEAL PORTION

BEVERAGES

CAPPUCCINO

1 cup made with 4 oz whole milk	5 cups made with 4 oz whole milk	1 cup made with 4 oz fat-free milk
80 calories	*400 calories*	*40 calories*

FAT-FREE MILK

1 cup	5 cups	1 cup
80 calories	*400 calories*	*80 calories*

LIGHT BEER (12 OZ BOTTLE)

1 bottle	4 bottles	1 bottle
100 calories	*400 calories*	*100 calories*

WINE (5 OZ GLASS)

1½ glasses	3⅓ glasses	1 glass
190 calories	*380 calories*	*120 calories*

BEER (12 OZ BOTTLE)

1 bottle	2½ bottles	1 bottle
150 calories	*380 calories*	*150 calories*

FIXES

1 Take the edge off your hunger by munching on raw vegetables or having a glass of vegetable juice before heading out.

2 Start your meal with soup to fill you up and help you eat fewer calories.

3 Always order dressing on the side to drizzle onto your salad. Chefs typically use a heavy hand that can add several hundred calories.

4 Avoid any dish that brags about its size with words like huge, large, grande, or jumbo.

5 Order your meat and fish grilled or broiled rather than sautéed or stir-fried. Grilling and broiling allow fat and calories to drip off.

6 Ask for a doggy bag at the same time as your meal is served, and put away excess food before you start eating.

7 To satisfy your sweet tooth, order just one dessert with enough spoons for everyone at the table.

8 Keep drinks simple— a glass of wine, light beer, or a calorie-free beverage—so that you have as many calories as possible for food.

DINER

Everything from burgers to salads and breakfasts to dinners

Diners are among the best bargains around, with very large portions at usually fair prices. Therein lies the problem—many diner dishes easily top 400 calories, and some are the equivalent of at least two 400-calorie meals! Plus, you're likely to be offered unlimited soft drink and bread basket refills, another source of extra calories. The good news is that diner menus usually have something for everyone, including sandwiches that are easy to split, salads with your choice of high- or lower-calorie dressings, plain grilled meats and fish, and several types of fresh fruit. As always, remember to ask for exactly what you want.

TYPICAL PORTION	400-CALORIE PORTION	MEAL PORTION

APPETIZERS

SMALL STUFFED MUSHROOMS (1")

8 mushrooms	6 mushrooms	2 mushrooms
550 calories	*410 calories*	*140 calories*

STUFFED POTATO SKINS

4 potato skins	6 potato skins	2 potato skins
280 calories	*420 calories*	*140 calories*

FRIED ZUCCHINI STICKS WITH MARINARA SAUCE

8 sticks (2 cups) + ¼ cup sauce	5 sticks (1¼ cups) + 2½ Tbsp sauce	2 sticks (½ cup) + 1 Tbsp sauce
620 calories	*420 calories*	*155 calories*

Skip the appetizers page of the menu. Most appetizers are extremely high in calories and otherwise low in nutrition.

Chicken Breast

2 small stuffed mushrooms
140

+

3 oz grilled chicken breast
140

+

Small salad
(1 cup lettuce +
½ medium tomato +
1 Tbsp honey mustard
dressing)
110

=

390
calories

★ *protein*
★ *fruits/veggies*

Split Pea Soup

1 cup split pea soup
190

·········· + ··········

4 saltine crackers
50

·········· + ··········

½ brownie + ¼ cup
vanilla ice cream
180

·········· = ··········

420
calories
★ *good fats*

Split pea
soup, bean soup,
and vegetarian
or meat-and-bean
chili are top sources
of fiber on the
diner menu.

TYPICAL PORTION	400-CALORIE PORTION	MEAL PORTION
SOUPS		
MATZO BALL SOUP		
1 bowl soup (1½ cups) + 3 matzo balls	1½ bowls soup (2¼ cups) + 5 matzo balls	1 bowl soup (1½ cups) + 1 matzo ball
260 calories	*430 calories*	*105 calories*
MANHATTAN CLAM CHOWDER		
1 bowl (1½ cups)	2 bowls (3 cups)	1 cup
200 calories	*400 calories*	*130 calories*
CHICKEN NOODLE SOUP		
1 bowl (1½ cups)	4 cups	1 bowl (1½ cups)
160 calories	*400 calories*	*160 calories*
SPLIT PEA SOUP		
1 bowl (1½ cups)	2 cups	1 cup
280 calories	*380 calories*	*190 calories*
CHILI with Cheddar cheese and sour cream		
1 bowl chili (2 cups) + 3 Tbsp Cheddar cheese + 2 Tbsp sour cream	¾ bowl chili (1½ cups) + 1 Tbsp Cheddar cheese + 1 Tbsp sour cream	1 cup chili + 1 Tbsp Cheddar cheese + 1 Tbsp sour cream
540 calories	*370 calories*	*260 calories*

TYPICAL PORTION	400-CALORIE PORTION	MEAL PORTION

SALADS

SMALL SALAD

1 cup lettuce + ½ medium tomato + 2 Tbsp honey mustard dressing	9 cups lettuce + 4½ medium tomatoes + 3 Tbsp honey mustard dressing	1 cup lettuce + ½ medium tomato + 1 Tbsp honey mustard dressing
180 calories	*415 calories*	*110 calories*

DIET PLATTER

1 cup fruit salad + 1 cup low-fat cottage cheese + 1 cup Jell-O + 2 slices tomato	1 platter	1 cup fruit salad + ½ cup low-fat cottage cheese + 2 slices tomato
430 calories	*430 calories*	*190 calories*

CHEF'S SALAD

4 cups romaine + 4 tomato wedges + 2 oz each turkey, ham, roast beef + 2 sliced eggs + ¼ cup sliced American cheese + 2 Tbsp sliced olives + 4 Tbsp ranch dressing	½ chef's salad	4 cups romaine + 4 tomato wedges + 1 oz each turkey, ham, roast beef + 1 egg + 1 tsp olive oil + 1 Tbsp balsamic vinegar
850 calories	*425 calories*	*260 calories*

Chef's Salad

2 stuffed potato skins
140

+

Chef's salad
(4 cups romaine
+ 4 tomato wedges +
1 oz each turkey, ham,
roast beef + 1 egg +
1 tsp olive oil +
1 Tbsp balsamic vinegar)
260

=

400
calories

★ *protein*
★ *fruits/veggies*

Greek Salad

1 small stuffed
mushroom
70

+

Greek salad (2 cups
romaine + 1 medium
tomato + 5 Greek
olives + 3 stuffed
grape leaves +
2 Tbsp crumbled
feta + 1 tsp oil +
vinegar to taste)
300

+

2 saltine crackers
25

=

395
calories

★ *good fats*
★ *fruits/veggies*

TYPICAL PORTION	400-CALORIE PORTION	MEAL PORTION
TUNA SALAD PLATTER (½-CUP SCOOP)		
2 scoops tuna salad (1 cup) + 2 lettuce leaves + 2 slices tomato	1½ scoops tuna salad (¾ cup) + 2 lettuce leaves + 2 slices tomato	1 scoop tuna salad (½ cup) + 2 lettuce leaves + 2 slices tomato
540 calories	*410 calories*	*280 calories*
GREEK SALAD		
2 cups romaine + 1 medium tomato + 5 Greek olives + 3 stuffed grape leaves + ¼ cup crumbled feta + 4 Tbsp Italian dressing	2⅓ cups romaine + 1 large tomato + 8 Greek olives + 4 stuffed grape leaves + 3 Tbsp crumbled feta + 1 Tbsp Italian dressing	2 cups romaine + 1 medium tomato + 5 Greek olives + 3 stuffed grape leaves + 2 Tbsp crumbed feta + 1 tsp oil + vinegar to taste
480 calories	*410 calories*	*300 calories*

Standard seasoned croutons will set you back about 25 calories for 2 tablespoons, or much more if the diner fries its own from leftover bread.

BREAKFAST AND
BRUNCH

Diners are as popular for breakfast and brunch as they are for lunch and dinner. Order à la carte for the most flexibility in putting together your 400-calorie meal.

BREAKFAST AND BRUNCH	CALORIES
½ grapefruit	50
½ cup scrambled Egg Beaters	60
1 slice whole wheat toast	70
2 pieces Canadian bacon	90
½ cantaloupe	90
1 cup orange juice	110
3 strips bacon	150
1 cup oatmeal	160
2 fried eggs	180
3 pancakes	180
1 Belgian waffle	190
2 scrambled eggs	200
¾ cup hash browns	200
3 sausage links	250
Blueberry muffin	360
3-egg cheese omelet	370

BREAKFAST AND BRUNCH CONDIMENTS	CALORIES
1 tsp jam	20
1 Tbsp fresh whipped cream	25
1 tsp butter	30
2 Tbsp maple syrup	100

Scrambled Egg Beaters and Toast

½ cup scrambled
Egg Beaters
60
+

2 slices
whole wheat toast
140
+

2 pats butter
60
+

2 tsp jam
40
+

1 cup orange juice
110
=

410
calories
★ *fruits/veggies*

Veggie Burger

Veggie burger
(1 whole wheat bun +
2 oz veggie burger
patty + 1 leaf lettuce +
1 slice tomato +
1 Tbsp ketchup)
245

+

2 Tbsp grilled onions
15

+

¼ cup cole slaw
90

+

¼ cup potato salad
75

=

425
calories
★ fiber

TYPICAL PORTION	400-CALORIE PORTION	MEAL PORTION

BURGERS AND SANDWICHES

HAM AND SWISS SANDWICH ON RYE

2 slices rye bread + 3 oz ham + 2 oz Swiss cheese + 1 leaf lettuce + 1 slice tomato + 2 Tbsp mayo	¾ sandwich	½ sandwich, no mayo + 1 tsp mustard
520 calories	*390 calories*	*165 calories*

VEGGIE BURGER

1 whole wheat bun + 2 oz veggie burger patty + 1 leaf lettuce + 1 slice tomato + 1 Tbsp ketchup	1⅔ burgers	1 burger
245 calories	*410 calories*	*245 calories*

TURKEY BURGER

1 white or wheat bun + 8 oz ground turkey patty + 1 leaf lettuce + 1 slice tomato + 1 Tbsp ketchup	¾ burger	½ burger
495 calories	*375 calories*	*250 calories*

TYPICAL PORTION	400-CALORIE PORTION	MEAL PORTION
LARGE CHICKEN CAESAR WRAP (10")		
10" wrap + ¼ cup lettuce + 3 oz grilled chicken + 2 Tbsp Parmesan + tomato + 2 Tbsp Caesar dressing	⅔ filled wrap	½ filled wrap, no dressing + 1 tsp olive oil + vinegar to taste
580 calories	*390 calories*	*250 calories*
TUNA MELT (½-CUP SCOOP)		
2 slices rye bread + 1 scoop tuna + 2 slices American cheese	¾ sandwich	½ sandwich
560 calories	*420 calories*	*280 calories*
OPEN-FACE ROAST BEEF SANDWICH AU JUS		
½ large roll + 8 oz roast beef	⅔ sandwich	½ sandwich
650 calories	*440 calories*	*325 calories*

To trim calories, choose lean meats like sirloin and pork tenderloin or lower-fat poultry such as skinless turkey and chicken breasts.

Hamburger

½ hamburger
380

+

2 French fries
30

=

410

calories

★ *protein*

TYPICAL PORTION	400-CALORIE PORTION	MEAL PORTION
GRILLED CHEESE SANDWICH		
2 slices white bread + 2 slices American cheese + 2 tsp unsalted butter	1¼ sandwiches	1 sandwich
340 calories	*425 calories*	*340 calories*
HAMBURGER		
1 hamburger bun + 8 oz lean beef patty + 1 leaf lettuce + 1 slice tomato + 1 Tbsp ketchup	½ hamburger	½ hamburger
775 calories	*380 calories*	*380 calories*
BBQ PORK SANDWICH		
1 hamburger bun + 4 oz BBQ pork + 1 leaf lettuce + 1 slice tomato	1 sandwich	1 sandwich
380 calories	*380 calories*	*380 calories*

TYPICAL PORTION	400-CALORIE PORTION	MEAL PORTION

SMOKED TURKEY CLUB

3 slices white bread + 3 oz smoked turkey + 3 strips bacon + 2 slices Swiss cheese + 2 leaves lettuce + 2 slices tomato + 3 Tbsp mayo	2 slices bread + 3 oz smoked turkey + 1 strip bacon + 1 slice Swiss cheese + 1 leaf lettuce + 1 slice tomato + 1 tsp mustard, no mayo	2 slices bread + 3 oz smoked turkey + 1 strip bacon + 1 slice Swiss cheese + 1 leaf lettuce + 1 slice tomato + 1 tsp mustard, no mayo
1,080 calories	*415 calories*	*415 calories*

ENTRÉES

ROASTED TURKEY BREAST WITH GRAVY

6 oz turkey + ¼ cup gravy	9 oz turkey + 6 Tbsp gravy	3 oz turkey + 2 Tbsp gravy
245 calories	*375 calories*	*125 calories*

GRILLED CHICKEN BREAST

6 oz	9 oz	3 oz
280 calories	*420 calories*	*140 calories*

CHOPPED SIRLOIN PATTY WITH GRAVY

6 oz sirloin + ¼ cup gravy	7 oz sirloin + ⅓ cup gravy	4 oz sirloin + 3 Tbsp gravy
340 calories	*400 calories*	*230 calories*

Smoked Turkey Club

Smoked turkey club
(2 slices bread +
3 oz smoked turkey +
1 slice Swiss + 1 strip
bacon + 1 leaf lettuce +
1 slice tomato +
1 tsp mustard,
no mayo)

=

415

calories

★ *protein*

Fillet of Sole

Broiled fillet of sole dinner (3 oz fillet of sole + 1 cup Manhattan clam chowder + 1 cup sautéed mixed vegetables + 1 medium roll)

=

420
calories

★ protein
★ fruits/veggies

TYPICAL PORTION	400-CALORIE PORTION	MEAL PORTION
HAM DINNER		
8 oz ham steak + 27 fries (1 cup) + 1 Tbsp ketchup + 1 cup lettuce + ½ medium tomato + 1 Tbsp honey mustard dressing	4 oz ham steak + 13 fries (½ cup) + 1 Tbsp ketchup + 1 cup lettuce + ½ medium tomato + ½ Tbsp honey mustard dressing	4 oz ham steak + 1 cup lettuce + ½ medium tomato + balsamic vinegar to taste
805 calories	*425 calories*	*170 calories*
BROILED FILLET OF SOLE DINNER		
6 oz fish + 1 cup Manhattan clam chowder + 1 cup sautéed mixed vegetables + 1 large baked potato with 2 Tbsp sour cream + 2 tsp butter	3 oz fish + 1 cup Manhattan clam chowder + 1 cup sautéed mixed vegetables + 1 medium roll	3 oz fish + 1 cup Manhattan clam chowder + 1 cup sautéed mixed vegetables + 1 medium roll
810 calories	*420 calories*	*420 calories*
MEAT LOAF (1", 3 OZ SLICE), NO GRAVY		
2½ slices	1 slice	1 slice
1,075 calories	*430 calories*	*430 calories*

TYPICAL PORTION	400-CALORIE PORTION	MEAL PORTION

SIDE DISHES

GRILLED ONIONS

½ cup	3⅓ cups	2 Tbsp
60 calories	*400 calories*	*15 calories*

SLICED TOMATOES

4 slices	100 slices	4 slices
15 calories	*375 calories*	*15 calories*

STEAMED GREEN BEANS

1 cup + 1 pat butter	10 cups	1 cup
70 calories	*400 calories*	*40 calories*

STEAMED BROCCOLI

1 cup + 2 Tbsp cheese sauce	8 cups, no sauce	1 cup
110 calories	*400 calories*	*50 calories*

POTATO SALAD

½ cup	1⅓ cups	¼ cup
150 calories	*400 calories*	*75 calories*

COLE SLAW

½ cup	1 cup	¼ cup
170 calories	*360 calories*	*85 calories*

Ham Dinner

Ham dinner (4 oz ham steak + 1 cup lettuce + ½ medium tomato + balsamic vinegar to taste)
170

+

½ cup rice pilaf
140

+

1 cup fruit salad
100

=

410
calories

★ *protein*
★ *fruits/veggies*

Sirloin Patty

4 oz chopped sirloin patty + 3 Tbsp gravy
230

························ **+** ························

¼ cup potato salad
75

························ **+** ························

1 cup sautéed mixed vegetables
90

························ **=** ························

395
calories

★ protein
★ fruits/veggies

	TYPICAL PORTION	400-CALORIE PORTION	MEAL PORTION
SAUTÉED MIXED VEGETABLES			
	1 cup	4½ cups	1 cup
	90 calories	*405 calories*	*90 calories*
MEDIUM DINNER ROLL			
	1 roll + 2 pats butter	2½ rolls + 5 pats butter	1 roll
	160 calories	*400 calories*	*100 calories*
PASTA			
	1 cup	1¾ cups	½ cup
	220 calories	*390 calories*	*110 calories*
RICE PILAF			
	1 cup	1½ cups	½ cup
	280 calories	*420 calories*	*140 calories*
LARGE BAKED POTATO (10½ OZ)			
	1 potato + 1 pat butter + 2 Tbsp sour cream	1 potato + 1 pat butter + 2 Tbsp sour cream	½ potato
	390 calories	*390 calories*	*140 calories*
BROWN RICE			
	1 cup	1¾ cups	⅔ cup
	220 calories	*390 calories*	*150 calories*

TYPICAL PORTION	400-CALORIE PORTION	MEAL PORTION

SWEET POTATO FRIES

24 fries + 2 Tbsp ketchup	30 fries + 2 Tbsp ketchup	12 fries + 1 Tbsp ketchup
330 calories	*400 calories*	*170 calories*

STEAK FRIES

1½ cups	1¼ cups	½ cup
510 calories	*425 calories*	*170 calories*

FRENCH FRIES

40 fries (1½ cups)	27 fries (1 cup)	13 fries (½ cup)
600 calories	*400 calories*	*200 calories*

DESSERTS

FRESH STRAWBERRIES

1 cup + 2 Tbsp whipped cream	4 cups + ½ cup whipped cream	1 cup
100 calories	*400 calories*	*50 calories*

CANTALOUPE

1 cup	8 cups	1 cup
50 calories	*400 calories*	*50 calories*

Belgian Waffle

1 Belgian waffle
190

+

1 tsp butter
30

+

2 Tbsp maple syrup
100

+

1 Tbsp fresh whipped cream
25

+

1 cup sliced strawberries
50

=

395

calories
★ *fruits/veggies*

TYPICAL PORTION	400-CALORIE PORTION	MEAL PORTION
FRUIT SALAD		
1 cup	4 cups	1 cup
100 calories	*400 calories*	*100 calories*
CHOCOLATE CREAM PIE (8", CUT INTO 6 SLICES)		
1 slice	1¼ slices	½ slice
340 calories	*425 calories*	*170 calories*
BROWNIE (3" SQUARE)		
1 brownie + ½ cup vanilla ice cream	1 brownie + ½ cup vanilla ice cream	½ brownie + ¼ cup vanilla ice cream
360 calories	*360 calories*	*180 calories*
STRAWBERRY CHEESECAKE (8", CUT INTO 8 SLICES)		
1 slice	1 slice	½ slice
360 calories	*360 calories*	*180 calories*
SUGAR COOKIE (3 OZ)		
1 cookie	1 cookie	½ cookie
410 calories	*410 calories*	*205 calories*
PECAN PIE (8", CUT INTO 6 SLICES)		
1 slice + ½ cup vanilla ice cream	½ slice + ½ cup vanilla ice cream	½ slice, no ice cream
710 calories	*425 calories*	*285 calories*

DRINK YOUR
CALORIES

Every dieter knows how easy it can be to pile on the calories with sugary sodas, but those aren't the only drink calories you need to be aware of.

1 cup black coffee or black or green tea	0 calories
1 Tbsp fat-free milk	5 calories
1 Tbsp whole milk	10 calories
1 tsp sugar	16 calories
1 Tbsp half-and-half	20 calories
1 tsp honey	20 calories
1 Tbsp flavored nondairy creamer	25 calories
1 cup tomato juice	40 calories
1 cup fat-free milk	80 calories
1 cup soy milk	110 calories
1 cup orange juice	110 calories
1 cup apple juice	110 calories
1 cup cranberry juice cocktail	140 calories
1 cup whole milk	150 calories

Diet Platter

Diet platter
(1 cup fruit salad +
½ cup low-fat
cottage cheese +
2 slices tomato)
190

+

½ sugar cookie
205

=

395

calories

★ *fruits/veggies*

Pecan Pie

1 cup
sliced strawberries
50

.... + ...

1 glass fat-free milk
80

.... + ...

½ slice pecan pie,
no ice cream
285

.... = ...

415
calories

★ *good fats*
★ *fruits/veggies*

TYPICAL PORTION	400-CALORIE PORTION	MEAL PORTION

BEVERAGES

SOFT DRINKS (16 OZ GLASS)

TYPICAL PORTION	400-CALORIE PORTION	MEAL PORTION
1 glass	2⅓ glasses	Unlimited diet soft drinks
170 calories	*400 calories*	*0 calories*

COFFEE

TYPICAL PORTION	400-CALORIE PORTION	MEAL PORTION
1 cup + 2 Tbsp half-and-half + 2 tsp sugar	6 cups with ¾ cup (12 Tbsp) half-and-half + ¼ cup (12 tsp) sugar	1 cup + 2 Tbsp whole milk + calorie-free sweetener
70 calories	*420 calories*	*20 calories*

FAT-FREE MILK (8 OZ GLASS)

TYPICAL PORTION	400-CALORIE PORTION	MEAL PORTION
1 glass	5 glasses	1 glass
80 calories	*400 calories*	*80 calories*

FIXES

1 Read through the entire menu before deciding what to order. Then be sure to pick enough veggies and fruit, with smaller portions of grain and protein foods.

2 If you have a choice of cooking methods, such as fried or broiled, choose the lower-fat methods. Go for broiled, grilled, and steamed, and say no to fried or pan-fried.

3 You may need to order "deluxe" to get lettuce and tomato on your burger or sandwich; deluxe dishes also come with fries. Ask if you can swap the fries for a side salad or extra veggies.

4 To keep burger calories under control, order a leaner meat like turkey, chicken, or even ostrich or bison; add bulk with freebie vegetables like lettuce and tomato; and leave half your bun on the plate.

5 Order wisely if you select a "dinner" that includes side dishes. A salad with dressing on the side, a broth- or tomato-based soup, and cooked vegetables usually are lower-calorie picks than potatoes or grain dishes.

Even if your coffee is served with little cups of half-and-half, don't be shy about asking for a small pitcher of milk instead.

ITALIAN

Southern Italian fare is especially popular

Italian restaurants are known for serving generous amounts of food, which easily can undo your best 400-calorie efforts. People tend to eat more calories when portions are larger, according to research at Cornell and Penn State. So use visual cues and other 400-calorie tools to fill your plate with the right amount of food. In general, if your pasta portion is no bigger than your fist, your protein portion is smaller than your palm, and vegetables take up at least half your plate, you will be well on your way to a 400-calorie meal.

TYPICAL PORTION	400-CALORIE PORTION	MEAL PORTION

APPETIZERS

PEPPERONCINI

¼ cup	10 cups	¼ cup
10 calories	400 calories	10 calories

PROSCIUTTO

6 thin slices	24 thin slices	3 thin slices
100 calories	400 calories	50 calories

PEPPERONI

10 slices	40 slices	5 slices
100 calories	400 calories	50 calories

KALAMATA OLIVES

10 olives	40 olives	5 olives
100 calories	400 calories	50 calories

ITALIAN BREAD, MEDIUM (½"-THICK SLICE)

6 slices	8 slices	1 slice
300 calories	400 calories	50 calories

HONEYDEW SLICE, SMALL (1" THICK), WRAPPED IN PROSCIUTTO

1 slice melon + 2 slices prosciutto	4½ slices melon + 9 slices prosciutto	1 slice melon + 1 slice prosciutto
90 calories	405 calories	60 calories

Appetizer Platter

2 stuffed mushrooms
140

+

1 slice honeydew wrapped in 1 slice prosciutto
60

+

3 pieces marinated artichoke heart
90

+

5 kalamata olives
50

+

Medium slice Italian bread
50

=

390
calories

★ *good fats*
★ *fruits/veggies*

Fried Calamari and Antipasti

½ cup fried calamari
130

········ **+** ········

5 slices pepperoni
50

········ **+** ········

1 oz provolone cheese
100

········ **+** ········

5 kalamata olives
50

········ **+** ········

5 steamed mussels
70

········ **=** ········

400
calories

★ protein
★ good fats

TYPICAL PORTION	400-CALORIE PORTION	MEAL PORTION
MARINATED ARTICHOKE HEARTS, cut into quarters		
6 pieces	13 pieces	3 pieces
180 calories	*390 calories*	*90 calories*
PROVOLONE CHEESE		
4 oz	4 oz	1 oz
400 calories	*400 calories*	*100 calories*
FRIED CALAMARI		
1½ cups	1½ cups	½ cup
400 calories	*400 calories*	*130 calories*
STEAMED MUSSELS		
25 mussels	30 mussels	10 mussels
340 calories	*410 calories*	*140 calories*
MOZZARELLA STICKS		
10 sticks + ½ cup marinara sauce	4 sticks + 6 Tbsp marinara sauce	2 sticks + 3 Tbsp marinara sauce
870 calories	*390 calories*	*195 calories*
BRUSCHETTA, MEDIUM (½" x 2")		
3 pieces	2 pieces	1 piece
620 calories	*410 calories*	*210 calories*
GARLIC BREAD, MEDIUM (2" SLICE)		
1 slice	2 slices	1 slice
210 calories	*420 calories*	*210 calories*

TYPICAL PORTION	400-CALORIE PORTION	MEAL PORTION

SOUPS

MINESTRONE SOUP

1 bowl (1½ cups)	2 bowls (3 cups)	1 cup
200 calories	*400 calories*	*130 calories*

PASTA E FAGIOLI SOUP

1 bowl (1½ cups)	1½ bowls (2¼ cups)	1 cup
250 calories	*375 calories*	*165 calories*

SALADS

FRESH MOZZARELLA (½ OZ SLICES)
with basil, tomato, olive oil

6 slices cheese + 6 basil leaves + 6 tomato slices + 1 Tbsp olive oil	6 slices cheese + 6 basil leaves + 6 tomato slices + 1 Tbsp olive oil	2 slices cheese + 2 basil leaves + 2 tomato slices + 1 tsp olive oil
380 calories	*380 calories*	*130 calories*

GARDEN SIDE SALAD

1 cup salad + ¼ cup Italian dressing	1⅓ cups salad + ⅓ cup Italian dressing	1 cup salad + 1 Tbsp Italian dressing
290 calories	*385 calories*	*160 calories*

Soup and Salad

1 cup
pasta e fagioli soup
165

+

1 cup garden side
salad + 1 Tbsp
Italian dressing
160

+

Medium slice Italian
bread
50

=

375

calories

★ *fiber*
★ *good fats*
★ *fruits/veggies*

Mozzarella Salad and Pizza

Fresh mozzarella salad
(2 slices cheese +
2 basil leaves +
2 tomato slices +
1 tsp olive oil)
130

.... + ...

½ slice vegetable and
feta deep-dish pizza
270

.... = ...

400
calories
★ *good fats*

TYPICAL PORTION	400-CALORIE PORTION	MEAL PORTION

PIZZA

VEGETABLE AND FETA DEEP-DISH PIZZA (14", CUT INTO 8 SLICES)

1 slice	¾ slice	½ slice
540 calories	*400 calories*	*270 calories*

MEDITERRANEAN MULTIGRAIN FLATBREAD PIZZA (10", CUT INTO 6 SLICES)

2 slices	2⅔ slices	2 slices
300 calories	*400 calories*	*300 calories*

ENTRÉES

SHRIMP SCAMPI

1½ cups	3¾ cups	¾ cup
160 calories	*400 calories*	*80 calories*

PASTA BOLOGNESE

1½ cups pasta with meat sauce	1½ cups pasta with meat sauce	¾ cup pasta with meat sauce
390 calories	*390 calories*	*195 calories*

PENNE ALLA VODKA

3 cups penne with sauce	2 cups penne with sauce	1 cup penne with sauce
630 calories	*420 calories*	*210 calories*

TYPICAL PORTION	400-CALORIE PORTION	MEAL PORTION
BAKED ZITI		
2½ cups	1 cup	½ cup
1,050 calories	*420 calories*	*210 calories*
EGGPLANT PARMIGIANA (4" x ½")		
2 slices	2 slices	1 slice
420 calories	*420 calories*	*210 calories*
LINGUINE WITH WHITE CLAM SAUCE		
2 cups linguine with sauce	1¼ cups linguine with sauce	⅔ cup linguine with sauce
660 calories	*410 calories*	*220 calories*
MEAT LASAGNA (4" x 4" PIECE)		
1 piece (1½ cups)	⅞ piece (1¼ cups)	½ piece (¾ cup)
480 calories	*420 calories*	*240 calories*
PASTA PRIMAVERA WITH SAUCE		
2 cups	1½ cups	1 cup
510 calories	*380 calories*	*255 calories*
VEAL SCALOPPINE		
8 oz	6 oz	4 oz
560 calories	*420 calories*	*280 calories*
TUSCAN STEAK		
8 oz steak + 1 cup spaghetti	4 oz steak + ⅔ cup spaghetti	3 oz steak + ½ cup spaghetti
880 calories	*410 calories*	*290 calories*

Tuscan Steak
3 oz Tuscan steak + ½ cup spaghetti
290
+
½ cup sautéed spinach
100
=
390
calories
★ *protein*

Linguine with Clam Sauce
⅔ cup linguine with white clam sauce
220
+
1 cup sautéed broccoli
90
+
¼ cup gelato
90
=
400
calories
★ *fruits/veggies*

Veal Scaloppine

4 oz veal scaloppine
280

+

Large steamed
artichoke, no butter
120

=

400
calories

★ *fiber*

TYPICAL PORTION	400-CALORIE PORTION	MEAL PORTION

SLICED CHICKEN, BROCCOLI, AND RIGATONI IN WHITE WINE SAUCE

6 oz chicken + 1 cup broccoli + 2 cups pasta with sauce	3 oz chicken + 1 cup broccoli + ½ cup pasta with sauce	2 oz chicken + 1 cup broccoli + ½ cup pasta with sauce
920 calories	*375 calories*	*300 calories*

FIND THE FAT

As a general rule, lighter-colored sauces have more fat and calories per ½ cup:

	CALORIES	FAT (g)
Red clam sauce	60	1
Marinara sauce	110	4
Vodka sauce	140	10
Meat sauce with Italian sausage	160	11
Alfredo sauce	180	13
White clam sauce	300	21
Pesto sauce	620	57

TYPICAL PORTION	400-CALORIE PORTION	MEAL PORTION
VEAL MARSALA		
6 oz	5 oz	4 oz
470 calories	*390 calories*	*310 calories*
CHICKEN MARSALA		
6 oz chicken + 1 cup pasta with sauce	4 oz chicken + ⅔ cup pasta with sauce	3 oz chicken + ½ cup pasta with sauce
620 calories	*420 calories*	*310 calories*
SPAGHETTI AND MEATBALLS		
2 cups spaghetti + 4 meatballs + 1 cup sauce	⅞ cup spaghetti + 1⅓ meatballs + ⅔ cup sauce	⅔ cup spaghetti + 1 meatball + ½ cup sauce
1,110 calories	*420 calories*	*320 calories*
CHEESE RAVIOLI WITH MARINARA SAUCE		
12 ravioli with sauce	7 ravioli with sauce	6 ravioli with sauce
660 calories	*385 calories*	*330 calories*
CHICKEN PARMESAN		
6 oz chicken + 3 cups pasta with sauce	2 oz chicken + ¾ cup pasta with sauce	2 oz chicken + ½ cup pasta with sauce
1,380 calories	*410 calories*	*350 calories*

Chicken Marsala

3 oz chicken Marsala + ½ cup pasta
310

+

1 biscotti
90

=

400
calories
★ *protein*

Meat Lasagna

½ piece meat lasagna
240

+

½ cup gelato
180

=

420
calories

Chicken Scaloppine

3 oz chicken scaloppine + ½ cup pasta
370

·················· + ··················

5 asparagus spears + 1 tsp lemon sauce
35

·················· = ··················

405
calories

★ protein
★ fruits/veggies

TYPICAL PORTION	400-CALORIE PORTION	MEAL PORTION
CHICKEN SCALOPPINE		
6 oz chicken + 1 cup pasta with sauce	3½ oz chicken + ½ cup pasta with sauce	3 oz chicken + ½ cup pasta with sauce
740 calories	*410 calories*	*370 calories*
CHICKEN FETTUCCINE ALFREDO		
6 oz chicken + 2½ cups pasta with sauce	2 oz chicken + ½ cup pasta with sauce	2 oz chicken + ½ cup pasta with sauce
1,410 calories	*380 calories*	*380 calories*

SIDE DISHES

STEAMED ASPARAGUS WITH LEMON SAUCE		
20 asparagus spears + ¼ cup lemon sauce	27 spears + ⅞ cup sauce	5 spears + 1 tsp sauce
310 calories	*410 calories*	*35 calories*
POLENTA		
1 cup	2½ cups	½ cup
160 calories	*400 calories*	*80 calories*
SAUTÉED BROCCOLI		
2 cups	4½ cups	1 cup
180 calories	*405 calories*	*90 calories*

TYPICAL PORTION	400-CALORIE PORTION	MEAL PORTION
SAUTÉED SPINACH		
2 cups	2 cups	½ cup
400 calories	*400 calories*	*100 calories*
STUFFED ARTICHOKE		
1 artichoke	1 artichoke	¼ artichoke
400 calories	*400 calories*	*100 calories*
STEAMED ARTICHOKE		
1 large artichoke + ¼ cup melted lemon butter	2 large artichokes + 2 Tbsp melted lemon butter	1 large artichoke, no butter
520 calories	*420 calories*	*120 calories*

À LA CARTE SAUCES AND PASTAS

RED CLAM SAUCE		
1 cup	3⅓ cups	½ cup
120 calories	*400 calories*	*60 calories*
MARINARA SAUCE		
1 cup	1¾ cups	½ cup
220 calories	*385 calories*	*110 calories*
VODKA SAUCE		
1 cup	1½ cups	½ cup
280 calories	*420 calories*	*140 calories*

Penne alla Vodka

1 cup penne alla vodka
210

+

¼ stuffed artichoke
100

+

Medium slice Italian bread
50

+

1 cup sliced strawberries drizzled with balsamic vinegar
50

=

410
calories
★ *fruits/veggies*

Pasta Primavera

1 small slice honeydew melon + 1 slice prosciutto
60

.... + ...

1 cup pasta primavera with sauce
255

.... + ...

1 glass prosecco
110

.... = ...

425

calories

★ *fruits/veggies*

TYPICAL PORTION	400-CALORIE PORTION	MEAL PORTION
MEAT SAUCE WITH ITALIAN SAUSAGE		
1 cup	1⅓ cups	½ cup
320 calories	*430 calories*	*160 calories*
WHITE CLAM SAUCE		
1 cup	⅔ cup	½ cup
600 calories	*400 calories*	*300 calories*

CARB WATCH

Some carb dishes are more dense in calories than others. Limit yourself to one or maybe two selections in order to keep your meal balanced and within the 400-calorie range.

Medium slice Italian bread	50 calories
½ cup polenta	80 calories
½ cup spaghetti	110 calories
½ cup macaroni	110 calories
½ cup meat tortellini	125 calories
2 ounces thin pizza crust (standard slice)	200 calories
Medium slice garlic bread	210 calories
4 ounces pizza crust (standard slice)	400 calories

TYPICAL PORTION	400-CALORIE PORTION	MEAL PORTION
SPAGHETTI		
1 cup	1¾ cups	½ cup
220 calories	*385 calories*	*110 calories*
CHEESE RAVIOLI		
6 ravioli	12 ravioli	6 ravioli
195 calories	*390 calories*	*195 calories*
MEAT TORTELLINI		
1 cup	1½ cups	1 cup
250 calories	*375 calories*	*250 calories*
CHEESE TORTELLINI		
1 cup	1½ cups	1 cup
260 calories	*390 calories*	*260 calories*
LOBSTER RAVIOLI		
8 ravioli	5½ ravioli	4 ravioli
580 calories	*400 calories*	*290 calories*

DESSERTS

STRAWBERRIES, sliced and drizzled with balsamic vinegar		
1 cup	8 cups	1 cup
50 calories	*420 calories*	*50 calories*
BISCOTTI (⅔ OZ)		
4 biscotti	4 biscotti	2 biscotti
360 calories	*360 calories*	*180 calories*

Spaghetti and Meatballs

Spaghetti and meatballs
(⅔ cup spaghetti +
1 meatball +
½ cup sauce)
320

+

1 cup sautéed broccoli
90

=

410
calories

★ *protein*
★ *fruits/veggies*

Tiramisu

⅔ square tiramisu

=

400

calories

	TYPICAL PORTION	400-CALORIE PORTION	MEAL PORTION
GELATO			
	1½ cups	1⅛ cups	½ cup
	540 calories	*400 calories*	*180 calories*
TIRAMISU (3" x 3" SQUARE)			
	1 square	⅔ square	½ square
	600 calories	*400 calories*	*300 calories*

BEVERAGES

	TYPICAL PORTION	400-CALORIE PORTION	MEAL PORTION
CAPPUCCINO			
	1 cup made with 4 oz whole milk	5 cups each made with 4 oz whole milk	1 cup made with 4 oz whole milk
	80 calories	*400 calories*	*80 calories*
PROSECCO (5 OZ GLASS)			
	1 glass	3⅔ glasses	1 glass
	110 calories	*405 calories*	*110 calories*
RED OR WHITE WINE (5 OZ GLASS)			
	1 glass	3½ glasses	1 glass
	120 calories	*420 calories*	*120 calories*
BEER (12 OZ BOTTLE)			
	1 bottle	2⅔ bottles	1 bottle
	150 calories	*400 calories*	*150 calories*

FIXES

1 Eat like an Italian—start your meal with a salad (with vinegar and a dash of oil rather than full-fat dressing), follow with a small portion of pasta, and then enjoy a simple entrée.

2 Stick with vegetable or fruit appetizers rather than using all your calories on fat-filled fare such as mozzarella sticks and other fried foods. If the appetizer menu falls short, check out the side dishes and desserts for additional options.

3 Put together your own combination of sauce, pasta, and protein (beef, veal, pork, seafood, or beans) so that you can better judge the portion size of each.

4 Ask your waitperson about the size of dishes and the number of people they serve. Many Italian restaurants provide family-size portions to be shared by three or four people.

5 Request a lunch-, appetizer-, or half-size portion of a main dish. You'll still have plenty of food, even enough to share or bring home leftovers.

6 Order cappuccino for dessert. Calories in an 8-ounce cup range from 40 for cappuccino made with fat-free milk to 80 for a drink made with whole milk.

Lobster Ravioli

4 lobster ravioli
290

+

½ cup marinara sauce
110

=

400
calories

MEXICAN

Everything in a tortilla, and more

Mexican food has the potential to be among the healthiest, with its whole grain corn tortillas, good fats–rich avocado, abundance of fresh salads and grilled vegetables, and sensible protein portions. But unlimited chips are standard; portions generally are huge, with three or even four 400-calorie items on the plate; high-fat, high-calorie toppings like cheese, sour cream, and guacamole are plentiful; and blended drinks have a meal's worth of calories. Mexican menus offer a lot of flexibility, however, if you order off the à la carte list to create your own 400-calorie meal.

| TYPICAL PORTION | 400-CALORIE PORTION | MEAL PORTION |

APPETIZERS AND SOUPS

BEEF NACHOS

8 nachos	3 nachos	1 nacho
1,150 calories	*420 calories*	*140 calories*

CHEESE QUESADILLA, LARGE (10"), topped with guacamole, sour cream, and salsa

1 quesadilla + ¼ cup each guacamole, sour cream, salsa	2½ wedges (⅓ quesadilla) + 2 Tbsp each guacamole, sour cream, salsa	1 wedge (⅛ quesadilla) + ½ Tbsp each guacamole, sour cream, salsa
1,200 calories	*430 calories*	*150 calories*

BLACK BEAN SOUP

1 bowl (1½ cups)	2¾ cups	1 cup
220 calories	*400 calories*	*150 calories*

TORTILLA SOUP

1 bowl (1½ cups)	2 cups	1 cup
300 calories	*400 calories*	*200 calories*

TORTILLA CHIPS WITH QUESO CHEESE DIP

20 chips + 1 cup dip	10 chips + ½ cup dip	5 chips + ¼ cup dip
920 calories	*460 calories*	*230 calories*

Cheese Quesadilla

1 wedge +
½ Tbsp each
guacamole,
sour cream, salsa
150

+

1 large
chicken enchilada
230

=

380
calories
★ *good fats*

Fish Taco

1 cup black bean soup
150

····················· + ·····················

1 fried fish taco with
cabbage, pico de gallo
250

····················· = ·····················

400
calories
★ *fiber*

TYPICAL PORTION	400-CALORIE PORTION	MEAL PORTION
CHEESE QUESADILLA, SMALL (7")		
1 quesadilla	¾ quesadilla	½ quesadilla
550 calories	*410 calories*	*275 calories*
TORTILLA CHIPS WITH GUACAMOLE		
60 chips + 1 cup guacamole	20 chips + ⅓ cup guacamole	20 chips + ⅓ cup guacamole
1,200 calories	*400 calories*	*400 calories*

1-2-3-400 CALORIE
MEXICAN

Mexican restaurant menus are packed with à la carte choices that make putting together a balanced meal easier and a lot of fun. And the 1-2-3-400 calorie system is perfect for filling your plate.

1. First, pile half your plate with lettuce, tomato, salsa, and grilled veggies.
2. Next, divide the remaining half into three sections and fill two of these with rice, a medium flour tortilla, or two corn tortillas.
3. Finally, fill the last section with steak, chicken, pork, fish, or beans as your protein.

TYPICAL PORTION	400-CALORIE PORTION	MEAL PORTION

ENTRÉES

SHRIMP TACO with shrimp, lettuce, tomato, salsa in a soft corn tortilla

3 tacos	2 tacos	1 taco
600 calories	*400 calories*	*200 calories*

BEAN AND CHEESE BURRITO, LARGE (ABOUT 5" x 3")

1 burrito	½ burrito	¼ burrito
840 calories	*420 calories*	*210 calories*

BEEF EMPANADA (3")

5 empanadas	2 empanadas	1 empanada
1,050 calories	*420 calories*	*220 calories*

CHICKEN ENCHILADA, LARGE (ABOUT 6" x 2")

1 enchilada	1¾ enchiladas	1 enchilada
230 calories	*400 calories*	*230 calories*

BEEF BURRITO WITH SOUR CREAM, LARGE (ABOUT 5" x 3")

1 burrito + 2 Tbsp sour cream	⅖ burrito + 2 tsp sour cream	¼ burrito + ½ Tbsp sour cream
960 calories	*380 calories*	*240 calories*

FRIED FISH TACO with cabbage, pico de gallo

1 taco	1½ tacos	1 taco
250 calories	*375 calories*	*250 calories*

Bean and Cheese Burrito

¼ large bean and cheese burrito
210

+

1 cup tortilla soup
200

=

410
calories

★ *protein*
★ *fiber*

Steak Taco

1 soft steak taco
with grilled veggies,
rice, beans, guacamole,
pico de gallo,
sour cream
310

·············· + ··············

1 bottle light beer
100

·············· = ··············

410
calories
★ *good fats*

TYPICAL PORTION	400-CALORIE PORTION	MEAL PORTION
CHICKEN FLAUTA WITH QUESO, LARGE (ABOUT 7" x 1")		
4 flautas + ½ cup queso	1½ flautas + 3 Tbsp queso	1 flauta + 2 Tbsp queso
1,070 calories	*400 calories*	*270 calories*
SOFT STEAK TACO with grilled veggies, rice, beans, guacamole, pico de gallo, sour cream		
4 tacos	1⅓ tacos	1 taco
1,240 calories	*415 calories*	*310 calories*
SHRIMP SALAD		
1½ cups lettuce + ½ cup tomato + ½ cup shrimp + 2 Tbsp cheese + 2 Tbsp salsa + 2 Tbsp tortilla strips + 4 Tbsp vinaigrette dressing	1 salad + 2 Tbsp vinaigrette dressing	1 salad, no dressing
520 calories	*430 calories*	*320 calories*
BEEF AND CHEESE ENCHILADA, SMALL (ABOUT 6" x 2")		
3 enchiladas	1⅓ enchiladas	1 enchilada
960 calories	*425 calories*	*320 calories*
PORK TAMALE (ABOUT 2" x 4")		
1 tamale	1 tamale	1 tamale
370 calories	*370 calories*	*370 calories*

TYPICAL PORTION	400-CALORIE PORTION	MEAL PORTION
CHILE RELLENO (ABOUT 2" x 4")		
1 chile relleno	½ chile relleno	½ chili relleno
740 calories	*370 calories*	*370 calories*
VEGETARIAN SOFT TACO		
4 tacos, each with 1 soft corn tortilla + ¼ cup refried beans + 2 Tbsp each salsa, guacamole + 1 Tbsp grated cheese	2 tacos	2 tacos
760 calories	*380 calories*	*380 calories*

Chicken Enchilada

8 tortilla chips
120

+

¼ cup salsa
20

+

2 Tbsp guacamole
40

+

1 large
chicken enchilada
230

=

410

calories
★ *good fats*

CONDIMENTS

Spice up your meal with these popular condiments. Most are extremely low in calories.

FOOD	PORTION	CALORIES
Jalapeño pepper	1	5
Chopped tomatoes	2 Tbsp	5
Shredded lettuce	½ cup	5
Pico de gallo	2 Tbsp	10
Salsa	2 Tbsp	10
Sliced olives	2 Tbsp	20
Guacamole	2 Tbsp	40
Sour cream	2 Tbsp	40

Taco Salad

Taco salad
(2 cups lettuce +
¼ cup each diced
tomato, ground beef,
refried beans +
2 Tbsp each shredded
cheese, salsa +
3 Tbsp guacamole +
10 tortilla chips)

·············· = ··············

400
calories

★ fiber
★ good fats
★ fruits/veggies

TYPICAL PORTION	400-CALORIE PORTION	MEAL PORTION
TACO OR TOSTADA SALAD		
2 cups lettuce + ½ cup each diced tomato, ground beef, refried beans, guacamole, sour cream + 2 Tbsp each shredded cheese, salsa + fried tortilla shell	2 cups lettuce + ¼ cup each diced tomato, ground beef, refried beans + 2 Tbsp each shredded cheese, salsa + 3 Tbsp guacamole + 10 tortilla chips	2 cups lettuce + ¼ cup each diced tomato, ground beef, refried beans + 2 Tbsp each shredded cheese, salsa + 3 Tbsp guacamole + 10 tortilla chips
1,600 calories	*400 calories*	*400 calories*
GRILLED VEGGIE BURRITO, LARGE (ABOUT 5" x 3"), with beans, cheese, lettuce, pico de gallo, and sour cream		
1 burrito	½ burrito	½ burrito
800 calories	*400 calories*	*400 calories*
STEAK TACO IN A CRISP TACO SHELL		
4 tacos, each with 1 shell + 2 oz steak + 2 Tbsp guacamole + 1 Tbsp green tomatillo salsa + 2 Tbsp lettuce	2 tacos	2 tacos
820 calories	*410 calories*	*410 calories*

TYPICAL PORTION	400-CALORIE PORTION	MEAL PORTION

CHICKEN FAJITA WITH SALSA AND GUACAMOLE

3 fajitas, each with 1 medium (7½") flour tortilla + 3 oz grilled chicken breast + ½ cup grilled peppers and onions + 2 Tbsp each salsa, guacamole	1 fajita	1 fajita
1,260 calories	*420 calories*	*420 calories*

À LA CARTE

CORN TORTILLA, SMALL (5–6")

1 tortilla	7 tortillas	1 tortilla
60 calories	*420 calories*	*60 calories*

FLOUR TORTILLA, SMALL (5–6")

1 tortilla	5 tortillas	1 tortilla
80 calories	*400 calories*	*80 calories*

BLACK BEANS

1 cup	2 cups	½ cup
200 calories	*400 calories*	*100 calories*

Chicken Fajita

Chicken fajita
(1 medium flour tortilla
+ 3 oz grilled chicken
breast + ½ cup grilled
peppers and onions +
2 Tbsp each salsa,
guacamole)

=

420
calories

★ *protein*
★ *good fats*

Pile your
fajita with grilled
veggies plus
virtually calorie-free
salsa, pico de
gallo, lettuce,
and tomato.

Veggie Fajita

1 cup grilled peppers and onions
200

·········· + ··········

½ cup black beans
100

·········· + ··········

1 small flour tortilla
80

·········· = ··········

380

calories

★ *fiber*
★ *fruits/veggies*

TYPICAL PORTION	400-CALORIE PORTION	MEAL PORTION
TORTILLA CHIPS		
20 chips	27 chips	8 chips
300 calories	*400 calories*	*120 calories*
GRILLED PORK TENDERLOIN		
6 oz	10 oz	3 oz
240 calories	*400 calories*	*120 calories*
FLOUR TORTILLA, MEDIUM (7½")		
1 tortilla	2¾ tortillas	1 tortilla
140 calories	*385 calories*	*140 calories*
CHILE CON CARNE		
1 cup	1½ cups	½ cup
280 calories	*420 calories*	*140 calories*
GRILLED CHICKEN BREAST		
6 oz	8½ oz	3 oz
280 calories	*400 calories*	*140 calories*
REFRIED BEANS		
1 cup	1⅓ cups	½ cup
300 calories	*400 calories*	*150 calories*
SPANISH RICE		
½ cup	1¼ cups	½ cup
160 calories	*400 calories*	*160 calories*

TYPICAL PORTION	400-CALORIE PORTION	MEAL PORTION
GRILLED FAJITA STEAK		
6 oz	7 oz	3 oz
340 calories	*400 calories*	*170 calories*
GRILLED PEPPERS AND ONIONS		
1 cup	2 cups	1 cup
200 calories	*400 calories*	*200 calories*
FLOUR TORTILLA, LARGE (10")		
1 tortilla	1¾ tortillas	1 tortilla
220 calories	*385 calories*	*220 calories*

Make-Your-Own Steak Salad

3 oz grilled fajita steak
170
+
½ cup refried beans
150
+
2 Tbsp chopped tomatoes
5
+
2 cups shredded lettuce
20
+
2 Tbsp pico de gallo
10
+
4 tortilla chips
60
=

415
calories
★ *protein*

FIND THE
FAT

The following terms on a Mexican menu are a surefire sign that a dish is oversized and very high in fat. Calorie counts over 1,000 are not unusual!

- Big
- Combo
- Crispy
- Grande
- Loaded
- Sampler
- Supreme
- Trio or tres
- Ultimate

Chips and Dip

6 oz frozen margarita
180

+

5 tortilla chips + ¼ cup queso dip
230

=

410
calories

TYPICAL PORTION	400-CALORIE PORTION	MEAL PORTION

DESSERTS

FLAN

½ cup	1⅓ cups	½ cup
150 calories	*400 calories*	*150 calories*

SOPAIPILLAS

5 sopaipillas	1½ sopaipillas	1 sopaipilla
1,350 calories	*405 calories*	*270 calories*

BEVERAGES

LIGHT BEER (12 OZ BOTTLE)

1 bottle	4 bottles	1 bottle
100 calories	*400 calories*	*100 calories*

MEXICAN BEER (12 OZ BOTTLE)

1 bottle	2½ bottles	1 bottle
150 calories	*375 calories*	*150 calories*

SANGRIA

1 cup	2½ cups	1 cup
160 calories	*400 calories*	*160 calories*

FROZEN MARGARITA (12 OZ GLASS)

1 glass	1 glass	½ glass
370 calories	*370 calories*	*180 calories*

FIXES

1 Take your portion of chips and then get rid of the basket. But there's no need to skimp on the salsa. Know your salsas—although red salsa looks hotter than green, usually green is spicier. Pico de gallo is made from fresh chopped vegetables.

2 Trim your dish by choosing just one high-fat, high-calorie topping, either cheese, sour cream, or guacamole, and just one grain, either tortilla or beans.

3 When you're dining with a group, order one meal for every three or four people and fill in with additional lower-calorie à la carte choices.

4 Swap out beef, chicken, pork, or fish for beans to create a vegetarian meal. Be sure to ask, however, if the beans are made with lard.

5 Ask if you can trade fried fish for grilled; grilled has more protein and fewer calories.

Guacamole usually is made from the creamy Hass (also known as California) avocado; Florida avocados tend to be more watery.

CHINESE

Cantonese, Szechuan, and other regional classics in a 400-calorie way

The calories in Chinese dishes depend on so many different factors—the amount of oil in the wok, the balance of meat and veggies, the amount served on the platter, the types and amount of sauces—that eating in a 400-calorie way often is guesswork, unless you have calorie info for your favorite place. That said, you can play it safe by ordering dishes with plenty of veggies and by taking sensible portions that are filling. You'll feel fullest from a combo of meat or other protein along with vegetables and just a small portion of rice.

| TYPICAL PORTION | 400-CALORIE PORTION | MEAL PORTION |

APPETIZERS

SHUMAI (SHRIMP DUMPLING)

| 5 dumplings | 17 dumplings | 3 dumplings |
| *120 calories* | *410 calories* | *70 calories* |

CHICKEN DUMPLING

| 6 dumplings | 14 dumplings | 3 dumplings |
| *170 calories* | *400 calories* | *85 calories* |

SPICY CHICKEN WINGS

| 8 wings | 8 wings | 3 wings |
| *400 calories* | *400 calories* | *150 calories* |

WONTON

| 6 wontons | 7½ wontons | 3 wontons |
| *320 calories* | *400 calories* | *160 calories* |

Ginger Chicken with Broccoli

1 cup hot and sour soup
80
+
3 shumai
70
+
1 cup ginger chicken with broccoli
160
+
½ cup white rice
100
=

410
calories
★ *protein*

Wontons are a smart appetizer choice for their combo of cabbage and other veggies plus lean meat.

Shrimp with Candied Walnuts

1 chicken lettuce wrap
160

··········· + ···········

1 cup shrimp with candied walnuts
250

··········· = ···········

410
calories

★ protein
★ good fats

	TYPICAL PORTION	400-CALORIE PORTION	MEAL PORTION
CHICKEN LETTUCE WRAP			
	4 wraps	2½ wraps	1 wrap
	640 calories	*400 calories*	*160 calories*
EGG ROLL (4" x 1")			
	2 egg rolls	2¼ egg rolls	1 egg roll
	350 calories	*390 calories*	*175 calories*
FRIED PORK DUMPLINGS WITH POT STICKER SAUCE			
	6 dumplings + ¼ cup sauce	6 dumplings + ¼ cup sauce	3 dumplings + 2 Tbsp sauce
	410 calories	*410 calories*	*205 calories*
SPARERIBS			
	8 spareribs	2½ spareribs	2 spareribs
	1,360 calories	*425 calories*	*340 calories*

FIND THE
FAT

These are a tip-off to fried, higher-fat, higher-calorie dishes:

- Crackling
- Crispy
- Deep-fried
- Diced
- Golden
- Sizzling

TYPICAL PORTION	400-CALORIE PORTION	MEAL PORTION

SOUPS

EGG DROP SOUP

1 bowl (1½ cups)	4 bowls (6 cups)	1 cup
100 calories	400 calories	70 calories

HOT AND SOUR SOUP

1 bowl (1½ cups)	3 bowls (4½ cups)	1 cup
120 calories	360 calories	80 calories

WONTON SOUP

1 bowl (1½ cups)	1¾ bowls (2⅔ cups)	1 cup
225 calories	390 calories	150 calories

ENTRÉES

GARLIC SHRIMP WITH VEGETABLES

4 cups	4 cups	1 cup
420 calories	420 calories	105 calories

STIR-FRIED BUDDHA'S FEAST

4 cups	3⅔ cups	1 cup
440 calories	400 calories	110 calories

SPICY GREEN BEANS

2 cups	3⅔ cups	1 cup
220 calories	400 calories	110 calories

Buddha's Feast

1 egg roll
175

+

1 cup stir-fried Buddha's Feast
110

+

½ cup brown rice
110

=

395

calories

★ fiber
★ fruits/veggies

Chicken Lo Mein

3 chicken dumplings
85
+
1 cup chicken lo mein
180
+
1 cup shrimp
with snow peas
140
=

405
calories

★ protein
★ fiber

TYPICAL PORTION	400-CALORIE PORTION	MEAL PORTION
STIR-FRIED EGGPLANT		
2 cups	1½ cups	½ cup
540 calories	*405 calories*	*135 calories*
SHRIMP WITH SNOW PEAS		
4 cups	2⅔ cups	1 cup
575 calories	*380 calories*	*145 calories*
VEGETABLE LO MEIN		
4 cups	1⅓ cups	½ cup
1,170 calories	*390 calories*	*150 calories*
GINGER CHICKEN WITH BROCCOLI		
4 cups	2½ cups	1 cup
650 calories	*400 calories*	*160 calories*
KUNG PAO CHICKEN		
3 cups	2¼ cups	1 cup
540 calories	*400 calories*	*180 calories*
CHICKEN LO MEIN		
4 cups	2¼ cups	1 cup
720 calories	*400 calories*	*180 calories*
PEPPER STEAK RICE BOWL ON BROWN RICE		
4 cups	2 cups	1 cup
790 calories	*395 calories*	*200 calories*

TYPICAL PORTION	400-CALORIE PORTION	MEAL PORTION
MA PO TOFU		
3 cups	2 cups	1 cup
630 calories	*420 calories*	*210 calories*
MU SHU PORK		
2 cups + 4 pancakes + ¼ cup sauce	⅞ cup + 1¾ pancakes + 5 tsp sauce	½ cup + 1 pancake + 1 Tbsp sauce
890 calories	*390 calories*	*220 calories*
SESAME CHICKEN		
3 cups	1¾ cups	1 cup
680 calories	*385 calories*	*230 calories*

Mu Shu Pork

½ cup mu shu pork +
1 pancake +
1 Tbsp sauce
220

+

½ cup vegetable lo mein
150

=

370
calories

BITE BY
BITE

Want to grab a couple bites of someone else's dish? Here's the calorie cost:

Buddha's feast	9 calories
Kung pao shrimp	16 calories
Sweet and sour pork	18 calories
Fried rice	18 calories
Beef and broccoli	21 calories
Egg roll	29 calories
General Tso's chicken	36 calories
Sparerib	42 calories

Beef and Broccoli

1 cup egg drop soup
70

+

1 cup
beef and broccoli
340

=

410
calories
★ *protein*

General Tso's Chicken

½ cup General Tso's
chicken
290

+

½ cup white rice
100

=

390
calories

	TYPICAL PORTION	400-CALORIE PORTION	MEAL PORTION
SPICY FISH			
	1½ cups	1¾ cups	1 cup
	340 calories	400 calories	230 calories
SHRIMP WITH CANDIED WALNUTS			
	1½ cups	1½ cups	1 cup
	380 calories	380 calories	250 calories
KUNG PAO SHRIMP			
	1½ cups	1½ cups	1 cup
	390 calories	390 calories	260 calories
ORANGE BEEF			
	3 cups	1½ cups	1 cup
	840 calories	420 calories	280 calories
SWEET AND SOUR PORK			
	3 cups	1½ cups	1 cup
	830 calories	410 calories	280 calories
GENERAL TSO'S CHICKEN			
	2 cups	⅔ cup	½ cup
	1,170 calories	390 calories	290 calories
BEEF AND BROCCOLI			
	3½ cups	1⅛ cups	1 cup
	1,170 calories	390 calories	340 calories

TYPICAL PORTION	400-CALORIE PORTION	MEAL PORTION

SIDE DISHES

WHITE RICE

1 cup	2 cups	½ cup
200 calories	*400 calories*	*100 calories*

BROWN RICE

1 cup	1¾ cups	½ cup
220 calories	*385 calories*	*110 calories*

FRIED RICE

1½ cups	1½ cups	½ cup
410 calories	*410 calories*	*140 calories*

VEGETABLE FRIED RICE

4 cups	1⅓ cups	½ cup
1,170 calories	*390 calories*	*150 calories*

CHICKEN FRIED RICE

1½ cups	1¼ cups	½ cup
500 calories	*420 calories*	*170 calories*

Sesame Chicken

1 cup sesame chicken
230
+
1 cup spicy green beans
110
+
¼ cup white rice
50
=

390
calories

★ *protein*
★ *good fats*
★ *fruits/veggies*

Use a Chinese teacup as a portion guide, with 1 teacup-size serving of rice and 2 for your main dish.

Wontons and Dumplings

3 wontons
160

.... + ...

3 fried pork dumplings + 2 Tbsp pot sticker sauce
205

.... + ...

1 fortune cookie
30

.... = ...

395
calories

★ *protein*

TYPICAL PORTION	400-CALORIE PORTION	MEAL PORTION

DESSERTS

FORTUNE COOKIE

1 cookie	13 cookies	1 cookie
30 calories	*390 calories*	*30 calories*

ORANGE WEDGES

2 wedges	53 wedges	8 wedges
15 calories	*400 calories*	*60 calories*

SPOT THE
SUGAR

Many classic Chinese sauces are full of added sugar.

- Char-siu
- Duck
- Hoisin
- Orange

- Oyster
- Peanut
- Plum
- Sweet and sour

FIXES

1 Start with a cup of soup to tame your appetite without too many calories.

2 Order dumplings steamed instead of fried to save up to 15 calories per dumpling.

3 Plan to share. Why use all your meal calories on one dish when you can take small amounts of several dishes?

4 Order one dish that is entirely vegetables, preferably steamed, and mix it into other dishes.

5 Leave as much sauce on the plate as you can. You need just a small amount for flavor, and Chinese sauces tend to pack in the calories because they can be high in fat and sugar.

Ma Po Tofu

1 cup ma po tofu
210

+

1 cup stir-fried
Buddha's Feast
110

+

8 orange wedges
60

+

1 fortune cookie
30

=

410
calories

★ *good fats*
★ *fruits/veggies*

JAPANESE

Mainly sushi plus a few main dish classics

Japanese cuisine deserves its reputation as one of the healthiest. Most traditional Japanese restaurants serve foods in modest portions, and many are prepared using very little fat. The picture is a little different in Americanized restaurants, where portions are larger and cooked with more oil. You may be able to hit the 400-calorie mark with a complete meal—usually miso soup, salad, main course, rice, and a vegetable—if you keep meal portions small. Or order à la carte, including sushi by the piece, for better control over calories.

| TYPICAL PORTION | 400-CALORIE PORTION | MEAL PORTION |

SUSHI AND SASHIMI

TUNA SASHIMI

TYPICAL PORTION	400-CALORIE PORTION	MEAL PORTION
1 piece	27 pieces	1 piece
15 calories	*405 calories*	*15 calories*

TORO (FATTY TUNA) SASHIMI

TYPICAL PORTION	400-CALORIE PORTION	MEAL PORTION
1 piece	20 pieces	1 piece
20 calories	*400 calories*	*20 calories*

BURI (YELLOWTAIL) SASHIMI

TYPICAL PORTION	400-CALORIE PORTION	MEAL PORTION
1 piece	20 pieces	1 piece
20 calories	*400 calories*	*20 calories*

EEL SASHIMI

TYPICAL PORTION	400-CALORIE PORTION	MEAL PORTION
1 piece	16 pieces	1 piece
25 calories	*400 calories*	*25 calories*

CUCUMBER ROLL

TYPICAL PORTION	400-CALORIE PORTION	MEAL PORTION
1 piece	13 pieces	1 piece
30 calories	*390 calories*	*30 calories*

CALIFORNIA ROLL

TYPICAL PORTION	400-CALORIE PORTION	MEAL PORTION
4 pieces	10 pieces	1 piece
160 calories	*400 calories*	*40 calories*

TUNA ROLL

TYPICAL PORTION	400-CALORIE PORTION	MEAL PORTION
4 pieces	10 pieces	1 piece
160 calories	*400 calories*	*40 calories*

Sashimi

4 pieces buri
(yellowtail) sashimi
80

+

4 pieces toro
(fatty tuna) sashimi
80

+

4 pieces eel sashimi
100

+

½ cup Japanese rice
120

=

380
calories

★ *protein*
★ *good fats*

Cucumber, California, and Futomaki Rolls

1 cup cucumber salad
30

+

4 pieces California roll
160

+

4 pieces futomaki
(vegetarian roll)
200

=

390
calories

★ good fats
★ fruits/veggies

The seaweeds wrapped around sushi and used in salads are rich in beta-carotene and folate, as well as several vital minerals.

	TYPICAL PORTION	400-CALORIE PORTION	MEAL PORTION
SEA DRAGON ROLL (eel, avocado, cucumber)			
	4 pieces	10 pieces	1 piece
	160 calories	*400 calories*	*40 calories*
TORO (FATTY TUNA) NIGIRI SUSHI			
	1 piece	8 pieces	1 piece
	50 calories	*400 calories*	*50 calories*
PHILADELPHIA ROLL (cream cheese, smoked salmon, cucumber)			
	4 pieces	8 pieces	1 piece
	200 calories	*400 calories*	*50 calories*
FUTOMAKI (vegetarian roll)			
	4 pieces	8 pieces	1 piece
	200 calories	*400 calories*	*50 calories*
SPICY SALMON ROLL			
	4 pieces	8 pieces	1 piece
	200 calories	*400 calories*	*50 calories*
ANAGO (EEL) NIGIRI SUSHI			
	1 piece	7 pieces	1 piece
	60 calories	*420 calories*	*60 calories*
EBI (SHRIMP) NIGIRI SUSHI			
	1 piece	7 pieces	1 piece
	60 calories	*420 calories*	*60 calories*

TYPICAL PORTION	400-CALORIE PORTION	MEAL PORTION
TEMAKI (hand roll with rice and salmon)		
1 roll	3⅓ rolls	1 roll
120 calories	*400 calories*	*120 calories*
CATERPILLAR ROLL (avocado, eel, cucumber)		
1 roll	1¼ rolls	½ roll
330 calories	*410 calories*	*165 calories*

FIND THE
FAT

Japanese cuisine includes several options for heart-healthy good fats, but you'll need to manage portion sizes to keep calories under control.

FOOD	TYPE OF FAT	CALORIES/OZ
Edamame (soybeans)	Monounsaturated fatty acids	38
Yellowtail	Omega-3 fatty acids	41
Mackerel	Omega-3 fatty acids	45
Avocado	Monounsaturated fatty acids	48
Salmon	Omega-3 fatty acids	51
Eel	Omega-3 fatty acids	67

Nigiri Sushi

2 pieces toro
(fatty tuna) nigiri sushi
100

+

1 piece anago (eel)
nigiri sushi
60

+

2 pieces ebi (shrimp)
nigiri sushi
120

+

1 piece
tempura banana
110

=

390
calories

Philadelphia and Tuna Rolls

1 cup shell-on edamame
100

·····+·····

4 pieces
Philadelphia roll
200

·····+·····

2 pieces tuna roll
80

·····=·····

380

calories
★ *good fats*

Beware of added sugar in carrot dressing and teriyaki sauce.

TYPICAL PORTION	400-CALORIE PORTION	MEAL PORTION

SOUPS AND SIDE DISHES

CUCUMBER SALAD

1 cup	13 cups	1 cup
30 calories	*390 calories*	*30 calories*

MISO SOUP

1 cup	10 cups	1 cup
40 calories	*400 calories*	*40 calories*

SIDE SALAD

1 cup lettuce + 1 Tbsp carrot dressing	8 cups lettuce + ½ cup carrot dressing	1 cup lettuce + 1 Tbsp carrot dressing
50 calories	*400 calories*	*50 calories*

STEAMED BROCCOLI

1 cup	8 cups	1 cup
50 calories	*400 calories*	*50 calories*

SEAWEED SALAD

1 cup	3½ cups	½ cup
120 calories	*420 calories*	*60 calories*

TEMPURA VEGETABLES

4 pieces	6 pieces	1 piece
270 calories	*405 calories*	*70 calories*

TYPICAL PORTION	400-CALORIE PORTION	MEAL PORTION
EDAMAME		
1 cup, shell-on	4 cups, shell-on	1 cup, shell-on
100 calories	*400 calories*	*100 calories*
JAPANESE RICE		
1 cup	1⅔ cups	½ cup
240 calories	*400 calories*	*120 calories*

ENTRÉES

BEEF NEGIMAKI		
8 pieces	11 pieces	4 pieces
300 calories	*410 calories*	*150 calories*
CHICKEN BREAST TERIYAKI		
6 oz	7¾ oz	3 oz
310 calories	*400 calories*	*155 calories*
UDON NOODLE BOWL		
2 cups	2¼ cups	1 cup
360 calories	*400 calories*	*180 calories*
SALMON TERIYAKI		
6 oz	6 oz	3 oz
420 calories	*420 calories*	*210 calories*

Salmon Teriyaki

1 cup miso soup
40
+
3 oz salmon teriyaki
210
+
1 cup steamed broccoli
50
+
½ cup Japanese rice
120
=

420
calories

★ protein
★ good fats
★ fruits/veggies

Chicken Teriyaki Bowl

2 cups sake
160
·····+·····
1½ cups chicken teriyaki bowl with vegetables, brown rice
240
·····=·····

400
calories

★ protein
★ fruits/veggies

	TYPICAL PORTION	400-CALORIE PORTION	MEAL PORTION
CHICKEN TERIYAKI BOWL with vegetables, brown rice			
	3 cups	2½ cups	1½ cups
	480 calories	*400 calories*	*240 calories*
STEAK TERIYAKI NOODLE BOWL with vegetables			
	3 cups	2 cups	1½ cups
	640 calories	*430 calories*	*320 calories*
SALMON TERIYAKI BOWL with vegetables, white rice			
	4 cups	2½ cups	2 cups
	650 calories	*410 calories*	*325 calories*

DESSERTS

	TYPICAL PORTION	400-CALORIE PORTION	MEAL PORTION
TEMPURA BANANA (1½" PIECE)			
	1 piece	4 pieces	1 piece
	110 calories	*440 calories*	*110 calories*
GREEN TEA ICE CREAM			
	½ cup	⅔ cup	¼ cup
	290 calories	*390 calories*	*145 calories*

BEVERAGES

	TYPICAL PORTION	400-CALORIE PORTION	MEAL PORTION
SAKE (2 OZ SAKE CUP)			
	2 sake cups	5 sake cups	2 sake cups
	160 calories	*400 calories*	*160 calories*

TYPICAL PORTION	400-CALORIE PORTION	MEAL PORTION

PLUM WINE (4 OZ GLASS)

1 glass	2¼ glasses	1 glass
180 calories	*400 calories*	*180 calories*

FIXES

1 For your 400-calorie sushi roll meal, eat about 8 standard-size pieces plus either miso soup or a vegetable salad to start.

2 Choose plain salmon or tuna sushi rolls rather than spicy. Spicy fillings are chopped and blended with mayo.

3 Leave some of the rice behind. Rice is the number one contributor of calories in a Japanese meal, and Japanese sushi rice is higher in calories because of added sugar. Or order your seafood as sashimi, pieces of raw fish served without rice.

4 Say no to tempura as a meal and limit yourself to just one piece. The fried coating adds plenty of calories to the naturally low-calorie vegetable or shrimp inside.

5 To add nutrition and balance to a sushi meal, look for vegetable dishes in the appetizer section of the menu. Many restaurants offer relatively low-calorie salads that are made from spinach, cucumber, or seaweed and seasoned with rice vinegar and a touch of sugar.

Beef Negimaki

1 glass plum wine
180

+

4 pieces beef negimaki
150

+

¼ cup Japanese rice
60

=

390
calories

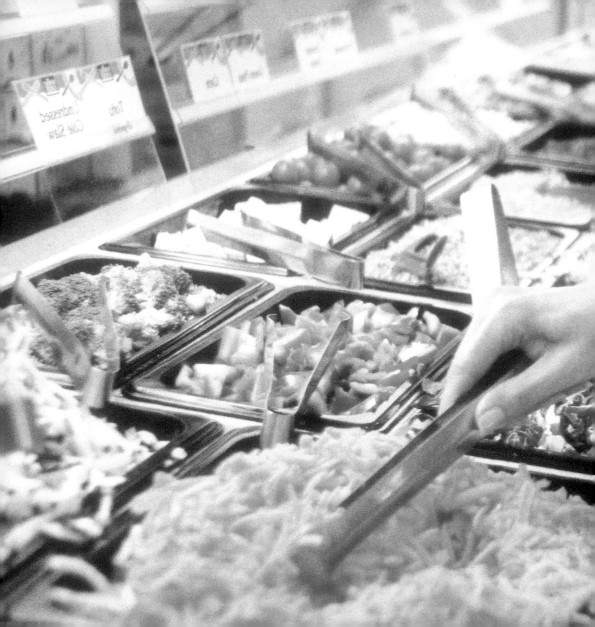

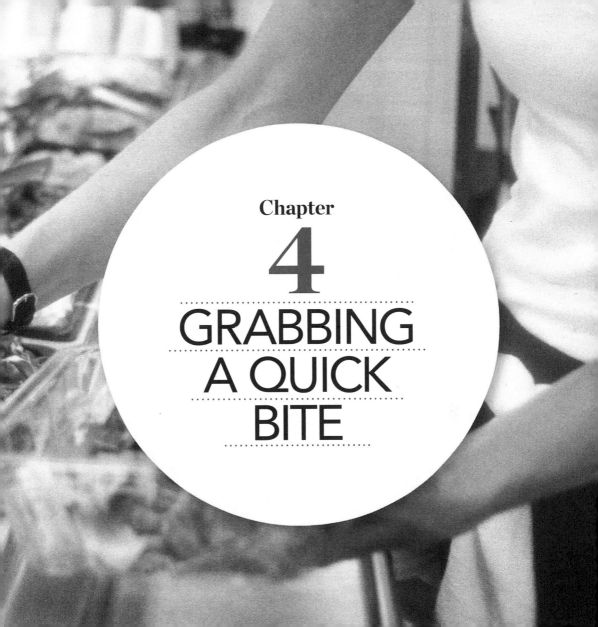

Chapter

4
GRABBING
A QUICK
BITE

FAST FOOD

The good news—a growing number of healthier choices

Food choices at fast-food restaurants are much improved, with an increasing number of choices for the nutrition-conscious. Still, you'll find very few whole wheat bread and bun choices, not many fiber-rich legumes, and a somewhat limited choice of veggies and fruits. If you're craving a burger or sandwich, compare calories—posted on the restaurant menu, in a brochure, or on a Web site—so that you can pick the size that best fits into a 400-calorie meal.

TYPICAL PORTION	400-CALORIE PORTION	MEAL PORTION

BURGERS AND DOGS

CHILI CHEESE DOG ON A BUN (6")

1 chili cheese dog	1 chili cheese dog	½ chili cheese dog
430 calories	*430 calories*	*215 calories*

HAMBURGER with lettuce, tomato, pickle, onion, ketchup, and mustard on a bun

Double hamburger	Double hamburger	Single hamburger
420 calories	*420 calories*	*250 calories*

BURGER KING WHOPPER with lettuce, tomato, mayo, ketchup, pickles, and onions on a sesame seed bun

1 Whopper with mayo	¾ Whopper, no mayo	½ Whopper, no mayo
670 calories	*390 calories*	*260 calories*

VEGGIE BURGER with lettuce, tomato, ketchup, and mayo on a sesame seed bun

Veggie burger with cheese and mayo	Veggie burger with cheese, no mayo	Veggie burger, no cheese or mayo
450 calories	*370 calories*	*320 calories*

HOT DOG ON A BUN (6")

1 hot dog	1¼ hot dogs	1 hot dog
350 calories	*440 calories*	*350 calories*

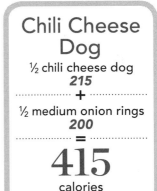

Hamburger and Fries

Single hamburger
250

··········· + ···········

½ small order fries
115

+

1 Tbsp ketchup
15

=

380
calories

Chili Cheese Dog

½ chili cheese dog
215

··········· + ···········

½ medium onion rings
200

=

415
calories

Grilled Chicken Sandwich

Grilled chicken sandwich with lettuce and tomato on ciabatta bread
360

.... **+** ....

1 Tbsp
light mayonnaise
40

.... **=** ....

400
calories

★ *protein*

TYPICAL PORTION	400-CALORIE PORTION	MEAL PORTION

CHICKEN AND FISH

KFC ORIGINAL RECIPE CHICKEN BREAST

1 breast	1¼ breasts	1 breast, no skin or breading
320 calories	*400 calories*	*150 calories*

MCDONALD'S CHICKEN MCNUGGETS

10 nuggets + 2 packets barbecue sauce	8 nuggets + 1 packet barbecue sauce	4 nuggets
560 calories	*420 calories*	*190 calories*

GRILLED CHICKEN SANDWICH with lettuce and tomato on ciabatta bread

1 sandwich, with mayo	1 sandwich, no mayo	1 sandwich, no mayo
470 calories	*360 calories*	*360 calories*

FISH FILLET SANDWICH ON A BUN

1 sandwich, with tartar sauce	1 sandwich, no tartar sauce	1 sandwich, no tartar sauce
560 calories	*380 calories*	*380 calories*

BREAKFAST
SANDWICHES

Most fast-food chains open their doors bright and early, making it that much easier to grab breakfast on the go. To keep within a 400-calorie framework with room for fruit or a beverage, think English muffin or flatbread rather than croissant or biscuit. Or enjoy a bowl of oatmeal with toppings.

Egg white and cheese on a wheat English muffin	260 calories
Egg white and turkey sausage flatbread sandwich	280 calories
Oatmeal with nuts and brown sugar	290 calories
Egg and cheese on an English muffin	300 calories
Egg white and cheese omelet on a 6" roll	320 calories
Plain bagel with 1 Tbsp cream cheese, 1 oz lox, thick slice tomato	385 calories
Chicken breakfast burrito	410 calories
Large ham, egg, and cheese croissant sandwich	410 calories
Bacon, egg, and cheese biscuit	420 calories
Egg on a bagel	530 calories

Whopper

½ Burger King Whopper, no mayo
260

················ + ················

1 value order Burger King Onion Rings
150

················ = ················

410
calories

Bite for bite, a hamburger has twice the protein of a hot dog.

Steak Tacos

1 Chipotle crispy steak taco
255

.... **+** ....

½ cup guacamole
160

.... **=** ....

415

calories

★ *good fats*

TYPICAL PORTION	400-CALORIE PORTION	MEAL PORTION

TACOS AND WRAPS

TACO BELL BEEF BURRITO SUPREME

1 burrito	1 burrito	½ burrito
420 calories	*420 calories*	*210 calories*

CHIPOTLE CRISPY STEAK TACO

2 crispy taco shells, each with 2 oz steak + 1 oz lettuce + 2 Tbsp grated cheese + 2 Tbsp tomato salsa + 2 Tbsp guacamole	1½ tacos	1 taco
510 calories	*380 calories*	*255 calories*

HONEY MUSTARD CHICKEN WRAP

1 wrap with crispy chicken	1½ wraps with grilled chicken	1 wrap with grilled chicken
330 calories	*390 calories*	*260 calories*

| TYPICAL PORTION | 400-CALORIE PORTION | MEAL PORTION |

SALADS

WENDY'S MANDARIN CHICKEN SALAD

TYPICAL PORTION	400-CALORIE PORTION	MEAL PORTION
1 salad (1½ cups) + 1 packet Crispy Noodles (⅓ cup) + 1 packet Roasted Almonds (¼ cup) + 1 packet Oriental Sesame Dressing (3 Tbsp)	1 salad (1½ cups) + 1 packet Roasted Almonds (¼ cup) + ½ packet Oriental Sesame Dressing (1½ Tbsp)	1 salad (1½ cups)
550 calories	*395 calories*	*180 calories*

KFC CHICKEN CAESAR SALAD

TYPICAL PORTION	400-CALORIE PORTION	MEAL PORTION
1 salad with crispy chicken (1½ cups) + 1 packet croutons + 1 packet KFC Creamy Parmesan Caesar Dressing (4 Tbsp)	1 salad with grilled chicken (1½ cups) + 1 packet croutons + ¼ packet KFC Creamy Parmesan Caesar Dressing (1 Tbsp)	1 salad with grilled chicken (1½ cups), no croutons or dressing
630 calories	*435 calories*	*200 calories*

Chicken Wrap

Honey mustard chicken wrap with grilled chicken
260

+

2 Tbsp barbecue sauce
50

+

1 cup side salad
40

+

2 Tbsp light Caesar dressing
30

=

380
calories

★ *protein*
★ *fruits/veggies*

Southwest Salad

McDonald's Premium
Southwest Salad with
Grilled Chicken +
1 packet Newman's
Own Low Fat Family
Recipe Italian Dressing

=

380

calories

★ protein
★ fruits/veggies

TYPICAL PORTION	400-CALORIE PORTION	MEAL PORTION
MCDONALD'S PREMIUM SOUTHWEST SALAD with Crispy Chicken		
1 salad (3 cups) + 1 packet Newman's Own Creamy Southwest Dressing (3 Tbsp)	1 salad (3 cups), no dressing	½ salad (1½ cups), no dressing
530 calories	*430 calories*	*215 calories*

SPOT THE
SUGAR

You expect to find lots of sugar in sugar-sweetened beverages and desserts, but other higher-sugar foods may surprise you.

2 Tbsp balsamic vinaigrette dressing	5 grams
2 Tbsp barbecue sauce	10 grams
1 packet fat-free French dressing	15 grams
1 packet Asian sesame vinaigrette dressing	17 grams
Small soft-serve ice cream cone	18 grams
Fruit and yogurt parfait	21 grams
Small (12 oz) cola	29 grams
Small (12 oz) vanilla shake	54 grams

TYPICAL PORTION	400-CALORIE PORTION	MEAL PORTION
PANERA FUJI APPLE WITH CHICKEN SALAD		
1 salad (3½ cups) + 1 packet Greek Dressing/Herb Vinaigrette (3 Tbsp) + 1 piece baguette (2 oz, 4")	½ salad (1¾ cups) + 1 packet Reduced Sugar Asian Sesame Vinaigrette (3 Tbsp) + ½ piece baguette (1 oz, 2")	½ salad (1¾ cups) + ½ packet Light Buttermilk Ranch Dressing
890 calories	*380 calories*	*300 calories*
MCDONALD'S PREMIUM SOUTHWEST SALAD with Grilled Chicken		
1 salad (3 cups) + 1 packet Newman's Own Creamy Southwest Dressing (3 Tbsp)	1 salad (3 cups) + 1 packet Newman's Own Low Fat Family Recipe Italian Dressing (3 Tbsp)	1 salad (3 cups), no dressing
420 calories	*380 calories*	*320 calories*
BAJA FRESH SAVORY ENSALATA WITH PORK CARNITAS		
1 salad (4 cups) + 2 packets Olive Oil Vinaigrette (6 Tbsp)	1 salad (4 cups) + 6 Tbsp salsa verde	1 salad (4 cups)
660 calories	*385 calories*	*370 calories*

Fish Sandwich
Fish fillet sandwich, no tartar sauce
·········· = ··········
380
calories

Veggie Burger

Burger King Veggie
Burger, no cheese,
no mayo
320

················· + ·················

1 Tbsp ketchup
15

················· + ·················

BK Fresh Apple Fries
with Caramel Sauce
65

················· = ·················

400
calories

★ *protein*
★ *fiber*
★ *fruits/veggies*

	TYPICAL PORTION	400-CALORIE PORTION	MEAL PORTION
CHIPOTLE SALAD			
	1 cup romaine + ½ cup each black beans, cilantro-lime rice, carnitas, and corn salsa + 4 Tbsp each cheese and vinaigrette	1 cup romaine + ½ cup each black beans, fajita veggies, cilantro-lime rice, tomato salsa + 4 Tbsp cheese	1 cup romaine + ½ cup each black beans, fajita veggies, cilantro-lime rice, tomato salsa + 4 Tbsp cheese
	890 calories	*400 calories*	*400 calories*

FRIES AND SIDES

KFC STEAMED GREEN BEANS

TYPICAL PORTION	400-CALORIE PORTION	MEAL PORTION
½ cup	10 cups	½ cup
20 calories	*400 calories*	*20 calories*

SALTINES

TYPICAL PORTION	400-CALORIE PORTION	MEAL PORTION
2 crackers	32 crackers	2 crackers
25 calories	*400 calories*	*25 calories*

SIDE SALAD

TYPICAL PORTION	400-CALORIE PORTION	MEAL PORTION
1 cup	10 cups	1 cup
40 calories	*400 calories*	*40 calories*

TYPICAL PORTION	400-CALORIE PORTION	MEAL PORTION
KFC CORN ON THE COB		
5½" ear	3 (5½") ears	3" ear
140 calories	*420 calories*	*70 calories*
KFC THREE-BEAN SALAD		
½ cup	2⅞ cups	½ cup
70 calories	*400 calories*	*70 calories*
MASHED POTATOES		
½ cup potatoes + 3 Tbsp gravy	1⅔ cups potatoes + 10 Tbsp gravy	½ cup potatoes, no gravy
120 calories	*400 calories*	*90 calories*
PANERA LOW-FAT VEGETARIAN BLACK BEAN SOUP		
1 bowl (1½ cups)	3½ cups	1 cup
170 calories	*385 calories*	*110 calories*
KFC 2" BISCUIT		
1 biscuit	2 biscuits	⅔ biscuit
180 calories	*360 calories*	*120 calories*
BURGER KING ONION RINGS		
1 large order (5 oz)	1 medium order (4 oz)	1 value order (1½ oz)
490 calories	*400 calories*	*150 calories*

Soup and Salad

1 cup Panera Low-Fat Vegetarian Black Bean Soup
110
+
½ Panera Fuji Apple with Chicken Salad
260
+
½ packet Light Buttermilk Ranch Dressing
40
=

410
calories

★ protein
★ fiber
★ fruits/veggies

Chili

1 bowl Wendy's chili +
2 saltine crackers +
3 Tbsp cheese

=

425

calories

★ protein
★ fiber

	TYPICAL PORTION	400-CALORIE PORTION	MEAL PORTION
GUACAMOLE			
	½ cup	1¼ cups	½ cup
	160 calories	400 calories	160 calories
FRENCH FRIES			
	1 large order (5.4 oz)	1 medium order (4.1 oz)	1 small order (2.5 oz)
	500 calories	380 calories	230 calories
LARGE BAKED POTATO (10 OZ)			
	1 potato with sour cream, chives, and buttery spread	1 potato with sour cream, chives, and buttery spread	1 potato
	370 calories	370 calories	270 calories
WENDY'S CHILI			
	1 bowl chili (1½ cups) + 2 saltine crackers + 3 Tbsp cheese	1 bowl chili (1½ cups) + 2 saltine crackers + 3 Tbsp cheese	1 cup chili + 2 saltine crackers + 3 Tbsp cheese
	425 calories	425 calories	320 calories

TYPICAL PORTION	400-CALORIE PORTION	MEAL PORTION

DESSERTS

BURGER KING FRESH APPLE FRIES WITH CARAMEL DIP

1 packet apples + 1 packet dip	6 packets apples + 6 packets dip	1 packet apples + 1 packet dip
65 calories	*390 calories*	*65 calories*

FRUIT CUP

1 cup	4 cups	1 cup
100 calories	*400 calories*	*100 calories*

MCDONALD'S VANILLA ICE CREAM CONE

1 cone	2⅔ cones	1 cone
150 calories	*400 calories*	*150 calories*

HOT FUDGE SUNDAE (¾ CUP)

1 sundae with peanuts	1 sundae with peanuts	1 sundae, no peanuts
375 calories	*375 calories*	*330 calories*

Vanilla Shake
1 small vanilla shake
=

420
calories

The ice cream at McDonald's is reduced fat, making it lower in calories.

Chicken Nuggets

4 McDonald's Chicken McNuggets
190

···· + ····

1 Tbsp ketchup
15

···· + ····

McDonald's Vanilla Ice Cream Cone
150

···· + ····

McDonald's Small Nonfat Cappuccino
60

···· = ····

415
calories

★ *good fats*

TYPICAL PORTION	400-CALORIE PORTION	MEAL PORTION

BEVERAGES

CAPPUCCINO

1 large caramel (20 oz)	1⅓ large caramel (27 oz)	1 small nonfat (12 oz)
290 calories	*390 calories*	*60 calories*

SHAKEN GREEN ICED TEA

1 large (24 oz)	3 large (72 oz)	1 small (12 oz)
130 calories	*390 calories*	*65 calories*

SWEET ICED TEA

1 large (32 oz)	1¾ large (56 oz)	1 small (12 oz)
230 calories	*400 calories*	*90 calories*

LOW-FAT MILK

1 carton (8 oz)	4 cartons (32 oz)	1 carton (8 oz)
100 calories	*400 calories*	*100 calories*

COLA

1 large (32 oz)	1⅓ large	1 small (12 fl oz)
310 calories	*410 calories*	*110 calories*

ORANGE JUICE

1 large (32 oz)	1 large (32 oz) + 1 small (12 oz)	1 small (12 oz)
250 calories	*390 calories*	*140 calories*

VANILLA SHAKE

1 large (32 oz)	1 small (12 oz)	1 small (12 oz)
1,110 calories	*420 calories*	*420 calories*

FIXES

1 Pick the smallest size possible, usually a single burger, regular-size hot dog, small fries, or small shake. Sizes differ, however, from chain to chain, a good argument for checking portion and calories before you order.

2 Take control of your order. Ask what comes standard to avoid surprisingly high-fat add-ons like special sauces. Ketchup and mustard are good lower-calorie options. To add more flavor and bulk, pile on the calorie-safe toppings like lettuce, tomato, sliced onions, and pickles. And if you have a choice of bread or bun, go for whole wheat or whole grain.

3 Choosing grilled chicken instead of crispy (fried) chicken on your salad saves more than 100 calories.

4 Always ask for low-fat or fat-free dressing, and use about half the packet. Even these can be pretty high in calories. For dipping or spreading, ketchup and plain mustard are best bets. Higher in calories are mayonnaise and mayo-based spreads and dressings (lots of oil), barbecue sauce (very sweet), and honey mustard sauce (sweet, plus made with oil).

5 Splitting an order with a friend or bringing half home are good ways to keep calories under control.

6 Say no to sour cream on your Mexican meal, and limit yourself to just one starchy item, either rice or a tortilla.

Mexican fast-food dishes tend to be higher in fiber from the whole grain corn tortillas, beans, and salsa.

DELI

The perfect lunch stop for sandwiches, soups, and salads

The menu at today's delis looks nothing like the delis of old. Now, you can choose from grilled meats and lower-fat deli favorites like ham and roast beef in addition to the more traditional, and higher-fat, salami and pastrami. Plus, your veggie choices have expanded from soggy iceberg lettuce leaves and pink tomato slices to a wide range of vegetable side dishes and salads. It still is important to make smart choices because portions are as big as ever and almost no full-size sandwich comes in under 500 calories.

TYPICAL PORTION	400-CALORIE PORTION	MEAL PORTION

SANDWICHES

GRILLED CHICKEN BREAST ON A WHOLE WHEAT ROLL

3 oz whole wheat roll + 3 oz chicken breast + 1 lettuce leaf + 1 slice tomato + ¼ cup roasted peppers + 2 Tbsp guacamole	1 sandwich	½ sandwich
440 calories	*440 calories*	*220 calories*

SUBWAY ITALIAN B.M.T. ON 9-GRAIN WHEAT BREAD (6")

1 sandwich	⅞ sandwich	½ sandwich
450 calories	*390 calories*	*225 calories*

SUBWAY VEGGIE DELITE ON 9-GRAIN WHEAT BREAD (6")

1 sandwich + 1 tsp olive oil blend	1½ sandwiches	1 sandwich, no olive oil blend
275 calories	*410 calories*	*235 calories*

Veggie Sandwich

Subway Veggie Delite on 9-grain bread, no olive oil blend (6")
235

+

1 cup Subway Golden Broccoli & Cheddar Soup
140

=

375
calories
★ *fiber*

Steak Sandwich

Quiznos Roadhouse Steak Sammie with dressing
250

.... **+** ....

1 bowl
Quiznos Tomato Basil Soup + 2 crackers
160

.... **=** ....

410
calories

TYPICAL PORTION	400-CALORIE PORTION	MEAL PORTION
GRILLED CHEESE WITH TOMATO		
2 slices white bread + 2 slices American cheese + 2 slices tomato + 2 Tbsp butter	⅞ sandwich	½ sandwich
470 calories	*410 calories*	*235 calories*
QUIZNOS ROADHOUSE STEAK SAMMIE WITH DRESSING		
1 Sammie	1⅔ Sammies	1 Sammie
250 calories	*420 calories*	*250 calories*
TUNA SALAD WRAP (5" x 3")		
10" flour tortilla + ½ cup tuna salad + 2 lettuce leaves + 2 slices tomato + 2 Tbsp sliced olives	¾ wrap	½ wrap
520 calories	*390 calories*	*260 calories*

	TYPICAL PORTION	400-CALORIE PORTION	MEAL PORTION
SALAD WRAP (6" x 3")			
13" whole wheat tortilla + 1 cup lettuce + 2 tomato slices + 2 Tbsp sliced olives + ¼ cup hummus + 2 Tbsp Italian dressing	¾ wrap		½ wrap
520 calories	*390 calories*		*260 calories*
GRILLED CHICKEN AND PESTO			
1 piece Italian bread (3") + 3 oz grilled chicken + 2 tomato slices + 2 Tbsp pesto	¾ sandwich		½ sandwich
540 calories	*405 calories*		*270 calories*

Tuna Salad Wrap

½ tuna salad wrap
260

+

¼ cup potato salad
75

+

¼ cup cole slaw
85

=

420
calories

★ *good fats*

Grilled chicken breast is almost entirely protein and is an excellent source of vitamin B$_6$ and the B vitamin niacin.

Grilled Chicken Breast on a Roll

½ grilled chicken breast sandwich on a whole wheat roll
220

+

1 cup small green salad + 1 tsp oil + vinegar
60

+

½ cup deli 3-bean salad
90

=

370
calories

★ *protein*
★ *fiber*
★ *good fats*
★ *fruits/veggies*

TYPICAL PORTION	400-CALORIE PORTION	MEAL PORTION
CHICKEN CAESAR WRAP (6" x 3")		
13" whole wheat tortilla + 4 oz chicken breast + ½ cup romaine + 2 Tbsp Parmesan + 2 Tbsp roasted peppers + 2 Tbsp Caesar dressing	⅗ wrap	½ wrap, no dressing
710 calories	*425 calories*	*275 calories*
DELI COMBO		
2 slices whole wheat bread + 2 oz each roast beef, turkey breast, Swiss cheese + 2 lettuce leaves + 2 slices tomato + 2 Tbsp mayo	½ sandwich	½ sandwich, no mayo
760 calories	*380 calories*	*280 calories*

TYPICAL PORTION	400-CALORIE PORTION	MEAL PORTION
GRILLED SALMON		
2 slices whole wheat bread + 4 oz grilled salmon + 2 lettuce leaves + 2 slices tomato + 2 Tbsp mayo + 1 tsp mustard	⅔ sandwich	½ sandwich
595 calories	*400 calories*	*300 calories*

Grilled Salmon on Whole Wheat

½ grilled salmon sandwich
300

+

½ cup deli 3-bean salad
90

=

390
calories

★ *protein*
★ *fiber*
★ *good fats*

SPOT THE SUGAR

What's to drink? If you're heading to the refrigerated case for a bottle of water or tea, read the label carefully. Enhanced teas, water beverages, and sports drinks often have sugars and calories in addition to their extra ingredients.

BEVERAGE	CALORIES PER CUP
Sparkling water, seltzer	0
Unsweetened iced tea	0
Water beverage	10–50
Sports drink	50–60
Iced tea	60–80

Turkey Sandwich on a Hard Roll

1 turkey sandwich on a hard roll, no cheese
320

·················· **+** ··················

¼ cup cole slaw
85

·················· **=** ··················

405

calories

★ *protein*

	TYPICAL PORTION	400-CALORIE PORTION	MEAL PORTION
HAM AND BRIE			
	2 slices thickly sliced country whole grain bread (1") + 4 oz ham + 2 oz Brie + 1 cup baby spinach + 1 tsp Dijon mustard	⅔ sandwich	½ sandwich
	605 calories	*400 calories*	*300 calories*
TURKEY ON A HARD ROLL			
	3½" hard roll + 4 oz deli turkey breast + 2 oz provolone cheese + 2 lettuce leaves + 2 slices tomato + 3 Tbsp roasted peppers + 1 tsp mustard	1 sandwich with 1 oz cheese	1 sandwich, no cheese
	520 calories	*420 calories*	*320 calories*
QUIZNOS PESTO TURKEY WITH CHEESE, DRESSING			
	1 Torpedo	1¼ Bullets	1 Bullet
	675 calories	*410 calories*	*330 calories*

TYPICAL PORTION	400-CALORIE PORTION	MEAL PORTION

ARBY'S ROAST BEEF SANDWICH ON A BUN (REGULAR SIZE)

1 sandwich	1 sandwich	1 sandwich
350 calories	*350 calories*	*350 calories*

PANERA BREAD FULL SMOKED HAM AND SWISS ON STONE-MILLED RYE BREAD

1 sandwich	½ sandwich	½ sandwich
700 calories	*350 calories*	*350 calories*

GRILLED VEGGIE WRAP (5" x 3")

10" flour tortilla + ½ cup marinated grilled vegetables (1 tennis ball) + 1 oz goat cheese (2 large marbles)	1⅛ wraps	1 wrap
355 calories	*400 calories*	*355 calories*

PANERA BREAD SMOKEHOUSE TURKEY PANINI ON THREE CHEESE BREAD

1 sandwich	½ sandwich	½ sandwich
720 calories	*360 calories*	*360 calories*

Veggie Wrap

Grilled veggie wrap
355

+

½ cup
cucumber-onion salad
50

=

405
calories

★ fiber
★ fruits/veggies

The 10" wrap on your wrap sandwich easily tops 200 calories, and extra-large wrappers can equal the calories in more than four slices of bread.

Deli Combo Sandwich

½ deli combo sandwich, no mayo
280

+

1 cup small green salad + 1 tsp oil + vinegar
60

+

¼ cup cole slaw
85

=

425
calories

★ protein
★ fruits/veggies

TYPICAL PORTION	400-CALORIE PORTION	MEAL PORTION

PREPARED SALADS

VINEGAR-MARINATED VEGETABLES

½ cup	10 cups	½ cup
20 calories	400 calories	20 calories

CUCUMBER-ONION SALAD

½ cup	4 cups	½ cup
50 calories	400 calories	50 calories

SMALL GREEN SALAD

1 cup + 2 Tbsp Italian dressing	4 cups + 4 Tbsp Italian dressing	1 cup + 1 tsp oil + vinegar to taste
100 calories	400 calories	60 calories

POTATO SALAD

½ cup	1⅓ cups	¼ cup
150 calories	400 calories	75 calories

COLE SLAW

½ cup	1¼ cups	¼ cup
170 calories	420 calories	85 calories

DELI 3-BEAN SALAD

½ cup	2¼ cups	½ cup
90 calories	400 calories	90 calories

CARROT-RAISIN SALAD

½ cup	1 cup	¼ cup
190 calories	380 calories	95 calories

TYPICAL PORTION	400-CALORIE PORTION	MEAL PORTION
FRUIT SALAD		
1 cup *100 calories*	4 cups *400 calories*	1 cup *100 calories*
MACARONI SALAD		
½ cup *220 calories*	⅞ cup *385 calories*	¼ cup *110 calories*

FIND THE
FAT

Fat is the wild card in sandwich fillings. Whether natural, added into a salad filling, or slathered onto a roll, mayonnaise, oil, and salad dressing add fat and calories.

FILLING	FAT (g/oz)
Roast beef	2
Steak	3
Hummus	3
Tuna, chicken, egg salad	5
Lower-fat cheese	6
Cheese	8
Italian salad dressing	8
Salami	10
Mayonnaise	22
Oil	28

Chicken Salad

½ cup deli 3-bean salad
90

+

½ cup chicken salad
250

+

½ cup marinated
vegetables
20

+

1 cup small green salad
+ 1 tsp oil + vinegar
60

=

420
calories

★ *protein*
★ *fiber*
★ *fruits/veggies*

Egg Salad Sandwich

½ cup egg salad
230

·············· + ··············

2 lettuce leaves +
2 slices tomato
20

·············· + ··············

¼ piece baguette
125

·············· + ··············

½ cup fruit salad
50

·············· = ··············

425
calories

★ *protein*
★ *fruits/veggies*

TYPICAL PORTION	400-CALORIE PORTION	MEAL PORTION
PASTA VEGETABLE SALAD		
½ cup	1⅓ cups	½ cup
150 calories	*400 calories*	*150 calories*
EGG SALAD		
½ cup	⅞ cup	½ cup
230 calories	*400 calories*	*230 calories*
CHICKEN SALAD		
½ cup	¾ cup	½ cup
250 calories	*375 calories*	*250 calories*
TUNA SALAD		
½ cup	¾ cup	½ cup
260 calories	*390 calories*	*260 calories*
HAM SALAD		
½ cup	¾ cup	½ cup
270 calories	*405 calories*	*270 calories*

TYPICAL PORTION	400-CALORIE PORTION	MEAL PORTION

SOUPS

MUSHROOM BARLEY SOUP

1 bowl (1½ cups)	4 bowls (6 cups)	1 cup
110 calories	*440 calories*	*70 calories*

QUIZNOS TOMATO BASIL SOUP

1 bowl (2 cups) + 2 crackers	2½ bowls (5 cups) + 5 crackers	1 cup + 1 cracker
160 calories	*400 calories*	*80 calories*

BROCCOLI CHEESE SOUP

1 bowl (1½ cups)	2⅔ bowls (4 cups)	1 cup
150 calories	*400 calories*	*100 calories*

CREAM OF TOMATO SOUP

1 bowl (1½ cups)	2⅔ bowls (4 cups)	1 cup
150 calories	*400 calories*	*100 calories*

CHICKEN NOODLE SOUP

1 bowl (1½ cups)	2½ bowls (3¾ cups)	1 cup
160 calories	*400 calories*	*110 calories*

Ham and Brie Sandwich

½ ham and Brie sandwich
300

+

1 cup cream of tomato soup
100

=

400
calories
★ *fiber*

Salad Wrap

½ salad wrap
260

.... **+** ....

1 cup minestrone soup
130

.... **=** ....

390
calories

★ *good fats*
★ *fruits/veggies*

Chicken Caesar Wrap

1 cup chicken noodle soup
110

.... **+** ....

½ chicken Caesar wrap, no dressing
275

.... **=** ....

385
calories

★ *protein*

TYPICAL PORTION	400-CALORIE PORTION	MEAL PORTION
BEEF BARLEY SOUP		
1 bowl (1½ cups)	2 bowls (3 cups)	1 cup
200 calories	*400 calories*	*130 calories*
MANHATTAN CLAM CHOWDER		
1 bowl (1½ cups)	2 bowls (3 cups)	1 cup
200 calories	*400 calories*	*130 calories*
MINESTRONE SOUP		
1 bowl (1½ cups)	2 bowls (3 cups)	1 cup
200 calories	*400 calories*	*130 calories*
SPLIT PEA WITH HAM SOUP		
1 bowl (1½ cups)	2 bowls (3 cups)	1 cup
200 calories	*400 calories*	*130 calories*
SUBWAY GOLDEN BROCCOLI & CHEDDAR SOUP		
1 bowl (1¼ cups)	2 bowls (2½ cups)	1 cup
180 calories	*360 calories*	*140 calories*
POTATO SOUP		
1 bowl (1½ cups)	1¾ bowls	1 cup
220 calories	*385 calories*	*150 calories*

BREAKFAST PASTRIES

TYPICAL PORTION	400-CALORIE PORTION	MEAL PORTION

BAGUETTE (6" PIECE)

1 piece	⅘ piece	¼ piece
500 calories	400 calories	125 calories

PLAIN BAGEL (4")

1 bagel + 1 Tbsp butter	1 bagel + 1 Tbsp butter	½ bagel, no butter
390 calories	390 calories	145 calories

BRAN MUFFIN (4 OZ)

1 muffin	1⅓ muffins	½ muffin
290 calories	390 calories	145 calories

BANANA BREAD (1" SLICE)

1 slice (⅛ loaf)	2 slices (¼ loaf)	1 slice (⅛ loaf)
180 calories	360 calories	180 calories

HARD ROLL (3½")

1 roll + 2 pats butter	2 rolls + 1 pat butter	1 roll + 1 pat butter
240 calories	375 calories	205 calories

SCONE (4 OZ)

1 scone	1 scone	½ scone
410 calories	410 calories	205 calories

Bagel

1 plain bagel
290

+

1 pat butter
30

+

1 cup fruit salad
100

=

420
calories

★ *fruits/veggies*

Surprisingly, a medium croissant is a lower-calorie pick. Most breakfast rolls and pastries weigh more and pack in more calories.

	TYPICAL PORTION	400-CALORIE PORTION	MEAL PORTION
BLUEBERRY MUFFIN (4 OZ)			
	1 muffin	⅞ muffin	½ muffin
	450 calories	390 calories	225 calories
MEDIUM CROISSANT (5")			
	1 croissant	1¾ croissants	1 croissant
	230 calories	400 calories	230 calories
CORN MUFFIN (4 OZ)			
	1 muffin	⅞ muffin	½ muffin
	470 calories	410 calories	235 calories

FIXES

1 Make "mustard, no mayo" your mantra. You'll save 100 calories for every tablespoon of mayo that isn't slathered onto your sandwich.

2 To up the fiber in the typically fiber-poor deli meal, request whole grain bread or wraps, order sandwiches with veggies, choose side salads made with beans, and enjoy fruit for dessert.

3 Take advantage of half-size soup and salad, soup and sandwich, or salad and sandwich specials. You can come close to 400 calories by picking a lower-calorie soup or salad and nixing mayo and other high-calorie spreads on your sandwich.

4 If a roll is bigger than your fist, it has too many calories.

5 Avoid salads that have a greasy sheen or white coating, sure signs that they're made with plenty of oil or mayo.

6 Switch to Alpine Lace or other lower-fat cheeses when available, and keep your portion to one regular or two thin slices.

7 Ask if any sandwich salads, such as tuna and chicken, are available with lower-fat mayo.

SALAD BAR

Enough choices for a meal or side dishes

A well-built salad can be a satisfying and slimming meal. Standard salad bar fare like vegetables, fruits, and beans are high in water and fiber to help fill you up. Sizing up portions is pretty easy using the standard serving spoons and scoops at most salad bars. As you build your salad, keep in mind the 1-2-3-400-Calorie approach—fill about half your plate with vegetables, a third with protein foods, and the remainder with grain foods. Watch the fat—if a salad looks oily or creamy, it may be packed with calories.

TYPICAL PORTION	400-CALORIE PORTION	MEAL PORTION

GREENS

MIXED BABY GREENS
1 cup	40 cups	1 cup
10 calories	400 calories	10 calories

ROMAINE
1 cup	40 cups	1 cup
10 calories	400 calories	10 calories

SPINACH LEAVES
1 cup	40 cups	1 cup
10 calories	400 calories	10 calories

ICEBERG LETTUCE
1 cup	40 cups	1 cup
10 calories	400 calories	10 calories

ARUGULA
1 cup	40 cups	1 cup
10 calories	400 calories	10 calories

Tortellini Salad

1 cup mixed baby greens
10
+
¼ cup chopped tomatoes
10
+
½ cup tortellini salad
190
+
¼ cup slivered turkey
60
+
2 Tbsp light ranch dressing
80
+
1 slice Italian bread
50
=
400
calories
★ fruits/veggies

Arugula Salad with Blue Cheese

1 cup arugula
10

.... **+** ....

2 Tbsp blue cheese
60

.... **+** ....

2 Tbsp chopped walnuts
100

.... **+** ....

¼ cup chopped egg
60

.... **+** ....

2 Tbsp bacon bits
70

.... **+** ....

2 Tbsp balsamic vinaigrette
90

.... **=** ....

390
calories

★ *good fats*
★ *fruits/veggies*

TYPICAL PORTION	400-CALORIE PORTION	MEAL PORTION

FRUITS AND VEGETABLES

ALFALFA SPROUTS

⅛ cup	50 cups	⅛ cup
1 calorie	*400 calories*	*1 calorie*

SHREDDED CABBAGE

¼ cup	20 cups	¼ cup
5 calories	*400 calories*	*5 calories*

SLICED CUCUMBER

¼ cup	20 cups	¼ cup
5 calories	*400 calories*	*5 calories*

CHOPPED CELERY

¼ cup	20 cups	¼ cup
5 calories	*400 calories*	*5 calories*

CHOPPED TOMATOES

¼ cup	10 cups	¼ cup
10 calories	*400 calories*	*10 calories*

SLICED MUSHROOMS

¼ cup	10 cups	¼ cup
10 calories	*400 calories*	*10 calories*

CHOPPED RED PEPPER

¼ cup	10 cups	¼ cup
10 calories	*400 calories*	*10 calories*

TYPICAL PORTION	400-CALORIE PORTION	MEAL PORTION
DICED BEETS		
¼ cup	6⅔ cups	¼ cup
15 calories	*400 calories*	*15 calories*

SALAD DRESSING

Salad dressing can make the difference between sensible and over-the-top calories. Choose light or fat-free whenever available, or sprinkle a bit of oil plus vinegar or lemon juice.

DRESSING	CALORIES PER 2 TBSP SCOOP	FAT (g)
Fat-free Italian	15	0
Fat-free ranch	30	0
Light Caesar	30	6
Light Italian	50	5
Olive oil (2 tsp)	80	9
Light ranch	80	7
Italian	85	8
Balsamic vinaigrette	90	8
Oil and vinegar (1 Tbsp each)	120	13
Blue cheese	140	15
Ranch	145	15
Honey mustard	160	15
Caesar	160	17

Beet Salad

1 cup
mixed baby greens
10
+

¼ cup diced beets
15
+

2 Tbsp
chopped walnuts
100
+

4 Tbsp crumbled
feta cheese
100
+

2 Tbsp balsamic
vinaigrette
90
+

½ cup couscous
90
=

405
calories
★ *good fats*
★ *fruits/veggies*

Tuna Salad

1 cup iceberg lettuce
10

+

½ cup tuna salad
260

+

1 piece cornbread
150

=

420

calories

★ protein
★ good fats
★ fruits/veggies

Skip the carrot-raisin salad and cole slaw—too many mayo calories—and pick grated carrots, raisins, and shredded cabbage instead.

TYPICAL PORTION	400-CALORIE PORTION	MEAL PORTION
GRATED CARROTS		
¼ cup	6⅔ cups	¼ cup
15 calories	400 calories	15 calories
RED ONION		
¼ cup	5 cups	¼ cup
20 calories	400 calories	20 calories

VINEGARS

Use virtually calorie-free vinegar to thin out your favorite regular dressing for close to the same flavor and fewer calories.

Apple cider	Tangy, usually little or no apple flavor
Balsamic	Heavy texture, dark color, sweet and sour flavor
Champagne	Light flavor with almost no sharpness
Distilled white	Harsh, best for cleaning chores
Malt	Robust flavor, usually served with fried fish
Red wine	Classic vinegar flavor, best for salad dressings
Rice	Mild flavor with almost no sharpness

TYPICAL PORTION	400-CALORIE PORTION	MEAL PORTION
BEAN SPROUTS		
¼ cup	5 cups	¼ cup
20 calories	*400 calories*	*20 calories*
MARINATED ARTICHOKE HEARTS		
¼ cup	3⅓ cups	¼ cup
30 calories	*400 calories*	*30 calories*
DICED AVOCADO		
¼ cup	1⅔ cups	¼ cup
60 calories	*400 calories*	*60 calories*

PREPARED SALADS

BEAN SALAD		
¼ cup	2¼ cups	¼ cup
45 calories	*405 calories*	*45 calories*
POTATO SALAD		
¼ cup	1⅓ cups	¼ cup
75 calories	*400 calories*	*75 calories*
PASTA SALAD		
¼ cup	1¼ cups	¼ cup
90 calories	*420 calories*	*90 calories*
COLE SLAW		
¼ cup	1¼ cups	¼ cup
85 calories	*425 calories*	*85 calories*

Chef's Salad with Pasta

1 cup romaine
10
+

¼ cup slivered turkey
60
+

¼ cup slivered ham
60
+

¼ cup pasta salad
90
+

4 Tbsp diced cheese
130
+

2 Tbsp light Italian dressing
50
=

400
calories

★ *protein*
★ *fruits/veggies*

Egg Salad

1 cup romaine
10

·············· **+** ··············

¼ cup egg salad
120

·············· **+** ··············

¼ cup diced avocado
60

·············· **+** ··············

2 Tbsp sunflower seeds
90

·············· **+** ··············

2 Tbsp fat-free
Italian dressing
15

·············· **+** ··············

Medium
whole wheat roll
100

·············· **=** ··············

395
calories

★ good fats
★ fruits/veggies

TYPICAL PORTION	400-CALORIE PORTION	MEAL PORTION
TORTELLINI SALAD		
¼ cup	1 cup	¼ cup
95 calories	*380 calories*	*95 calories*
CARROT RAISIN SALAD		
¼ cup	1 cup	¼ cup
100 calories	*400 calories*	*100 calories*
FRUIT SALAD		
1 cup	4 cups	1 cup
100 calories	*400 calories*	*100 calories*
MACARONI SALAD		
¼ cup	⅞ cup	¼ cup
110 calories	*385 calories*	*110 calories*
EGG SALAD		
¼ cup	⅞ cup	¼ cup
120 calories	*420 calories*	*120 calories*
TUNA SALAD		
¼ cup	¾ cup	¼ cup
130 calories	*390 calories*	*130 calories*
CHICKEN SALAD		
¼ cup	¾ cup	¼ cup
130 calories	*390 calories*	*130 calories*

TYPICAL PORTION	400-CALORIE PORTION	MEAL PORTION

PROTEINS

CHOPPED EGG WHITE

¼ cup	3⅓ cups	¼ cup
30 calories	400 calories	30 calories

GRATED MOZZARELLA CHEESE

2 Tbsp	1¼ cups	2 Tbsp
40 calories	400 calories	40 calories

TOFU CUBES

¼ cup	2½ cups	¼ cup
40 calories	400 calories	40 calories

KIDNEY BEANS

¼ cup	2 cups	¼ cup
50 calories	400 calories	50 calories

COTTAGE CHEESE

¼ cup	2 cups	¼ cup
50 calories	400 calories	50 calories

CRUMBLED FETA CHEESE

2 Tbsp	1 cup	2 Tbsp
50 calories	400 calories	50 calories

CHICKEN BREAST CHUNKS

¼ cup	1⅔ cups	¼ cup
60 calories	400 calories	60 calories

Chicken Pasta Salad

1 cup mixed
baby greens
10
+
½ cup macaroni
110
+
¼ cup chopped egg
60
+
½ cup chicken breast
chunks
120
+
2 Tbsp raisins
50
+
2 Tbsp light Caesar
dressing
30
=

380
calories

★ protein
★ fruits/veggies

Salad and Cottage Cheese Platter

½ cup bean salad
90

+

½ cup potato salad
150

+

½ cup cottage cheese
100

+

4 saltine crackers
50

=

390
calories

★ protein
★ fruits/veggies

TYPICAL PORTION	400-CALORIE PORTION	MEAL PORTION
SLIVERED TURKEY		
¼ cup *60 calories*	1⅔ cups *400 calories*	¼ cup *60 calories*
SLIVERED HAM		
¼ cup *60 calories*	1⅔ cups *400 calories*	¼ cup *60 calories*
CHOPPED EGG		
¼ cup *60 calories*	1⅔ cups *400 calories*	¼ cup *60 calories*
GRATED CHEDDAR CHEESE		
2 Tbsp *60 calories*	⅞ cup *420 calories*	2 Tbsp *60 calories*

Hard cheeses like Parmesan and Cheddar supply more calcium than softer cheeses like Brie.

TYPICAL PORTION	400-CALORIE PORTION	MEAL PORTION
BLUE CHEESE		
2 Tbsp	⅞ cup	2 Tbsp
60 calories	*420 calories*	*60 calories*
DICED JACK CHEESE		
2 Tbsp	¾ cup	2 Tbsp
65 calories	*390 calories*	*65 calories*
GARBANZO BEANS		
¼ cup	1½ cups	¼ cup
70 calories	*420 calories*	*70 calories*

TOPPINGS

TYPICAL PORTION	400-CALORIE PORTION	MEAL PORTION
SLICED OLIVES		
2 Tbsp	2½ cups	2 Tbsp
20 calories	*400 calories*	*20 calories*
GRATED PARMESAN		
2 Tbsp	1¼ cups	2 Tbsp
40 calories	*400 calories*	*40 calories*
RAISINS		
2 Tbsp	1 cup	2 Tbsp
50 calories	*400 calories*	*50 calories*
DRIED CRANBERRIES		
2 Tbsp	1 cup	2 Tbsp
50 calories	*400 calories*	*50 calories*

Mediterranean Salad

1 cup romaine
10

+

¼ cup kidney beans
50

+

½ cup garbanzo beans
140

+

2 Tbsp crumbled feta cheese
50

+

2 Tbsp light Italian dressing
50

+

Medium whole wheat roll
100

=

400
calories

★ *fiber*
★ *fruits/veggies*

Chinese Salad

1 cup spinach leaves
10

+

½ cup tofu cubes
80

+

2 Tbsp sliced almonds
70

+

2 Tbsp crispy Chinese noodles
70

+

½ cup brown rice
110

+

Balsamic vinegar +
2 tsp oil
80

=

420
calories

★ *fiber*
★ *good fats*
★ *fruits/veggies*

TYPICAL PORTION	400-CALORIE PORTION	MEAL PORTION
LARGE CROUTONS		
8 croutons	64 croutons	8 croutons
50 calories	*400 calories*	*50 calories*
BACON BITS		
2 Tbsp	¾ cup	2 Tbsp
70 calories	*420 calories*	*70 calories*
CRISPY CHINESE NOODLES		
2 Tbsp	¾ cup	2 Tbsp
70 calories	*420 calories*	*70 calories*
SLICED ALMONDS		
2 Tbsp	¾ cup	2 Tbsp
70 calories	*420 calories*	*70 calories*

Almonds have more vitamin E than other nuts, while walnuts are highest in omega-3 fatty acids.

TYPICAL PORTION	400-CALORIE PORTION	MEAL PORTION
SUNFLOWER SEEDS		
2 Tbsp	9 Tbsp	2 Tbsp
90 calories	*405 calories*	*90 calories*
CHOPPED WALNUTS		
2 Tbsp	½ cup	2 Tbsp
100 calories	*400 calories*	*100 calories*
CHOPPED PEANUTS		
2 Tbsp	7 Tbsp	2 Tbsp
110 calories	*385 calories*	*110 calories*

BREADS, CRACKERS, AND GRAINS

TYPICAL PORTION	400-CALORIE PORTION	MEAL PORTION
COUSCOUS		
¼ cup	2¼ cups	¼ cup
45 calories	*405 calories*	*45 calories*
SALTINES		
4 crackers (2 packets)	32 crackers (16 packets)	4 crackers (2 packets)
50 calories	*400 calories*	*50 calories*
ITALIAN BREAD (2" x ½" SLICE)		
1 slice	8 slices	1 slice
50 calories	*400 calories*	*50 calories*

Chicken Salad

1 cup fruit salad
100

+

½ cup chicken salad
260

+

1 slice Italian bread
50

=

410
calories

★ *protein*
★ *fruits/veggies*

Chicken and Cranberry Salad

1 cup mixed baby greens
10

+

¼ cup chicken breast chunks
60

+

2 Tbsp dried cranberries
50

+

2 Tbsp chopped peanuts
110

+

2 Tbsp fat-free ranch dressing
30

+

1 piece cornbread
150

=

410
calories

★ good fats
★ fruits/veggies

TYPICAL PORTION	400-CALORIE PORTION	MEAL PORTION
MACARONI		
¼ cup	1¾ cups	¼ cup
55 calories	*385 calories*	*55 calories*
BROWN RICE		
¼ cup	1¾ cups	¼ cup
55 calories	*385 calories*	*55 calories*
MEDIUM WHOLE WHEAT ROLL (1½ OZ)		
1 roll	4 rolls	1 roll
100 calories	*400 calories*	*100 calories*
CORNBREAD (2.5" SQUARE)		
1 piece	2⅔ pieces	1 piece
150 calories	*400 calories*	*150 calories*

The more colors in your salad, the more health-promoting phyto-chemicals.

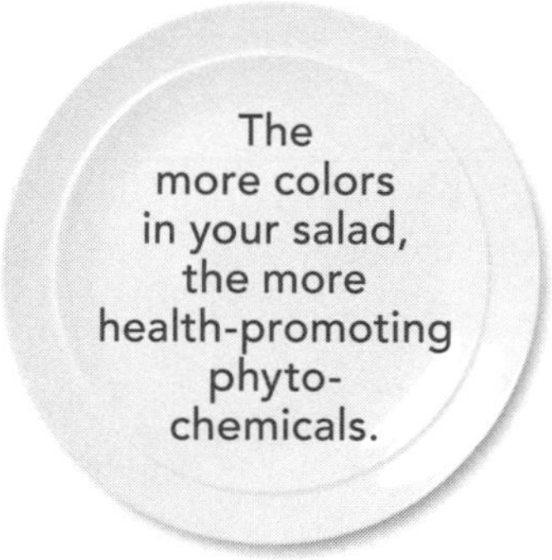

FIXES

1 Big calorie busters are prepared salads, cheese, and salad dressing. So if you're not being charged by weight, pile your plate high with plain veggies; they are filling and have very few calories.

2 To bulk up your salad without breaking the bank at a pay-by-the-pound salad bar, add items that don't weigh a lot, such as baby lettuce, alfalfa sprouts, shredded vegetables, and grated (rather than chunk) cheese.

3 For the best nutrition balance, your salad should be a combination of vegetables, protein, and a grain.

4 Decide between a roll or a scoop of a pasta, grain, or potato salad—they all supply similar nutrients.

5 Go for plain salad bar proteins like slivered or cubed turkey and ham, tuna chunks, tofu cubes, and cottage cheese rather than prepared salads for a lot of protein in relatively few calories.

6 Use salad bar spoons as a visual cue, with a flat spoon equaling 2 tablespoons and a rounded spoon equaling 4 tablespoons, or ¼ cup.

7 Dish up prepared salads with a slotted or perforated spoon so that calorie-rich dressing can drip off.

8 Put salad dressing in a small cup to dab onto your salad as you eat.

PIZZA

Popular pizzas plus classic pasta dishes

It is possible to stay within 400 calories at a pizza parlor, but it is harder to select a balanced meal because a slice of pizza leaves few extra calories to spare. One slice of a large (14″) traditional New York–style cheese pizza weighs in at about 320 calories, and that's before you add extra toppings. While a standard slice is not large enough to hold a star-worthy cup of veggies, ordering extra vegetables on your pizza adds nutritional value and makes your slice more satisfying and filling.

PIZZA

TYPICAL PORTION	400-CALORIE PORTION	MEAL PORTION

SMALL THIN-CRUST CHEESE PIZZA (10", CUT INTO 6 SLICES)

3 slices	3 slices	1½ slices
400 calories	400 calories	200 calories

INDIVIDUAL FOUR-CHEESE DEEP-DISH PIZZA (6", CUT INTO 4 SLICES)

4 slices	⅘ slice	½ slice
1,920 calories	380 calories	240 calories

PERSONAL PAN VEGETABLE PIZZA (6", CUT INTO 4 SLICES)

4 slices	3 slices	2 slices
550 calories	410 calories	275 calories

DEEP-DISH SPINACH PIZZA (12", CUT INTO 6 SLICES)

2 slices	1⅓ slices	1 slice
580 calories	390 calories	290 calories

LARGE CHICAGO-STYLE DOUBLE-CRUST DEEP-DISH PIZZA (14", CUT INTO 8 SLICES)

1 slice	½ slice	½ slice
580 calories	290 calories	290 calories

LARGE CHEESE PIZZA (14", CUT INTO 8 SLICES)

2 slices	1¼ slices	1 slice
640 calories	400 calories	320 calories

Cheese Pizza

1 slice large
cheese pizza
320

+

¼ cup mushrooms
on top
5

+

¼ cup sliced
bell peppers on top
5

+

Small salad
(1 cup lettuce +
½ tomato + 1 Tbsp
light Italian dressing)
45

=

375
calories
★ *fruits/veggies*

Broccoli-Chicken Pizza

1 slice broccoli pizza
335

.... **+** ....

¼ cup sliced grilled chicken breast on top
60

.... **=** ....

395

calories

★ *protein*

PIZZA DECONSTRUCTED

Many pizza shops allow you to customize your slice. Choose from these toppings:

TOPPING	CALORIES
¼ cup baby spinach leaves	0
¼ cup sliced bell pepper	5
¼ cup sliced mushrooms	5
1 large slice red onion	15
¼ cup broccoli	15
1 Tbsp Parmesan	20
2 Tbsp sliced olives	20
2 anchovies	20
¼ cup sliced ham	25
2 Tbsp marinara sauce	28
¼ cup pineapple	30
2 Tbsp mozzarella	40
4 slices pepperoni	40
1 slice bacon	45
¼ cup chicken breast strips	60
¼ cup ground beef	80
¼ cup sausage crumbles	100
1 slice crust only, 14" pie	200

TYPICAL PORTION	400-CALORIE PORTION	MEAL PORTION
LARGE BROCCOLI PIZZA (14", CUT INTO 8 SLICES)		
2 slices	1¼ slices	1 slice
670 calories	*420 calories*	*335 calories*
LARGE BBQ CHICKEN PIZZA (14", CUT INTO 8 SLICES)		
2 slices	1 slice	1 slice
760 calories	*380 calories*	*380 calories*
LARGE PEPPERONI PIZZA (14", CUT INTO 8 SLICES)		
2 slices	1 slice	1 slice
780 calories	*390 calories*	*390 calories*
LARGE DEEP-DISH PIZZA (14", CUT INTO 8 SLICES)		
2 slices	1 slice	1 slice
820 calories	*410 calories*	*410 calories*

Hawaiian Pizza

1 cup minestrone soup
130

+

1½ slices small
thin-crust cheese pizza
200

+

¼ cup sliced ham on top
25

+

¼ cup pineapple on top
30

=

385
calories

Ham is
lower in fat
and calories
than sausage,
ground meat,
or bacon.

Eggplant Parmigiana

¾ cup eggplant parmigiana
320

·············· + ··············

Small salad
(1 cup lettuce +
½ tomato + 1 Tbsp light
Italian dressing)
45

·············· = ··············

365
calories
★ *fruits/veggies*

TYPICAL PORTION	400-CALORIE PORTION	MEAL PORTION

PASTA

BAKED ZITI

2½ cups	1 cup	¾ cup
1,050 calories	*420 calories*	*320 calories*

SPAGHETTI AND MEATBALLS (2 OZ EACH)

2 cups spaghetti + 4 meatballs + 1 cup sauce	1 cup spaghetti + 1 meatball + ½ cup sauce	⅔ cup spaghetti + 1 meatball + ½ cup sauce
1,110 calories	*390 calories*	*320 calories*

EGGPLANT PARMIGIANA

1 cup	1 cup	¾ cup
420 calories	*420 calories*	*320 calories*

PASTA WITH MARINARA SAUCE

2 cups pasta + 1 cup sauce	1⅓ cups pasta + ½ cup sauce	1 cup pasta + ½ cup sauce
660 calories	*410 calories*	*330 calories*

CHEESE RAVIOLI WITH MARINARA SAUCE

12 ravioli + 1 cup sauce	7 ravioli + ⅝ cup sauce	6 ravioli + ½ cup sauce
660 calories	*400 calories*	*330 calories*

TYPICAL PORTION	400-CALORIE PORTION	MEAL PORTION

SOUP AND SALAD

SMALL SALAD

1 cup lettuce + ½ tomato + 2 Tbsp Italian dressing	3½ cups lettuce + 1¾ tomatoes + ½ cup Italian dressing	1 cup lettuce + ½ tomato + 1 Tbsp light Italian dressing
110 calories	*425 calories*	*45 calories*

MINESTRONE SOUP

1 bowl (1½ cups)	2 bowls (3 cups)	1 cup
200 calories	*400 calories*	*130 calories*

Baked Ziti

¾ cup baked ziti
320

+

1 bottle light beer
100

=

420
calories

Specialty cheese and cream sauces are higher in calories than traditional marinara or pizza sauce.

Deep-Dish Spinach Pie

1 slice deep-dish spinach pizza
290

+

1 glass red wine
120

=

410
calories

Personal Pizza

2 slices personal pan vegetable pizza
275

+

½ bottle cola
125

=

400
calories

TYPICAL PORTION	400-CALORIE PORTION	MEAL PORTION

BEVERAGES

LIGHT BEER (12 OZ BOTTLE)

1 bottle	4 bottles	1 bottle
100 calories	*400 calories*	*100 calories*

RED OR WHITE WINE (5 OZ GLASS)

1 glass	3½ glasses	1 glass
120 calories	*420 calories*	*120 calories*

COLA (20 OZ BOTTLE)

1 bottle	1½ bottles	½ bottle
250 calories	*375 calories*	*125 calories*

BEER (12 OZ BOTTLE)

1 bottle	2⅔ bottles	1 bottle
150 calories	*400 calories*	*150 calories*

The thicker the crust, the fewer calories to spare for toppings.

FIXES

1 Say no to almost anything "extra" like extra cheese, extra-thick crust, or an extra-large slice. Extra-thin crust, however, is a good idea because it's lower in calories, giving you room for more toppings and a side dish.

2 Stick with a slice from a medium-size (12") pizza. In most pizza shops, one sensibly topped slice falls well within your 400-calorie limit.

3 Take control of your toppings to customize your slice the way you want it. Vegetables always are a safe bet, as are lean meats like sliced chicken breast or sliced ham.

4 Jazz up your slice with pizza shop shaker toppings such as oregano, Italian spices, garlic powder, and spicy red-pepper flakes. They are calorie freebies.

5 Eat half the crust if deep-dish is your only option. It has up to twice the calories of thin crust. Thin crust and flatbread crust have about the same number of calories.

6 Use a napkin to blot off the extra oil from a greasy pizza slice, and save more than 100 calories.

VENDING MACHINE

Plenty of choices when the midafternoon slump hits

The vending machine is not the place to turn for a healthy balanced meal, even with the industry's efforts to improve the selection. So your goal is to make smart choices to keep your meal within the 400-calorie range while picking items that can fill you up and provide at least a bit of nutrition in the form of fiber or protein. Generally, you can choose a couple of different snacks—check out recommended portion sizes and their calories on the back of the pack—or enjoy just one snack if you're also having a drink with calories.

TYPICAL PORTION	400-CALORIE PORTION	MEAL PORTION

CHIPS, CRACKERS, AND PRETZELS

FRITOS ORIGINAL CORN CHIPS (3⅜ OZ BAG)

1 bag	¾ bag	¼ bag
560 calories	*420 calories*	*140 calories*

SUNCHIPS (1 OZ BAG)

15 chips (1 bag)	45 chips (3 bags)	15 chips (1 bag)
140 calories	*420 calories*	*140 calories*

ANDY CAPP'S HOT FRIES (1 OZ BAG)

50 fries (1 bag)	133 fries (2⅔ bags)	50 fries (1 bag)
150 calories	*400 calories*	*150 calories*

DORITOS NACHO CHEESE (1 OZ BAG)

11 chips (1 bag)	29 chips (2⅔ bags)	11 chips (1 bag)
150 calories	*400 calories*	*150 calories*

SNYDER'S OF HANOVER SOURDOUGH SPECIALS PRETZELS (1.65 OZ BAG)

8 pretzels (1 bag)	20 pretzels (2½ bags)	8 pretzels (1 bag)
160 calories	*400 calories*	*160 calories*

BAKED LAY'S POTATO CRISPS (1⅜ OZ BAG)

21 crisps (1 bag)	52 crisps (2½ bags)	21 crisps (1 bag)
160 calories	*400 calories*	*160 calories*

Chex Mix

1 bag Traditional Chex Mix
220

+

8 Snyder's of Hanover Sourdough Specials Pretzels
160

=

380

calories

Cheese and Chocolate

2 Reese's
Peanut Butter Cups
220

··············· **+** ···············

38 Cheez-It
Reduced Fat Crackers
190

··············· **=** ···············

410
calories
★ *good fats*

	TYPICAL PORTION	400-CALORIE PORTION	MEAL PORTION
FUNYUNS (1¼ OZ BAG)			
	16 pieces (1 bag)	36 pieces (2¼ bags)	16 pieces (1 bag)
	175 calories	*390 calories*	*175 calories*
CHEEZ-IT REDUCED FAT CRACKERS (1½ OZ BAG)			
	38 crackers (1 bag)	76 crackers (2 bags)	38 crackers (1 bag)
	190 calories	*380 calories*	*190 calories*
CHEDDAR GOLDFISH (1½ OZ BAG)			
	75 goldfish (1 bag)	150 goldfish (2 bags)	75 goldfish (1 bag)
	200 calories	*400 calories*	*200 calories*
WHEAT THINS TOASTED CHIPS (1½ OZ BAG)			
	21 chips (1 bag)	37 chips (1¾ bags)	21 chips (1 bag)
	220 calories	*385 calories*	*220 calories*
TRISCUIT ORIGINAL CRACKERS (1.94 OZ BAG)			
	12 crackers (1 bag)	20 crackers (1⅔ bags)	12 crackers (1 bag)
	240 calories	*400 calories*	*240 calories*
LAY'S POTATO CHIPS (1⅞ OZ BAG)			
	28 chips (1 bag)	42 chips (1½ bags)	28 chips (1 bag)
	280 calories	*420 calories*	*280 calories*

TYPICAL PORTION	400-CALORIE PORTION	MEAL PORTION

RITZ BITS PEANUT BUTTER (3 OZ BAG)

36 sandwiches (1 bag)	36 sandwiches (1 bag)	36 sandwiches (1 bag)
420 calories	*420 calories*	*420 calories*

CANDY

LIFE SAVERS (14-PIECE ROLL)

14 pieces (1 roll)	28 pieces (2 rolls)	1 piece ($\frac{1}{14}$ roll)
210 calories	*420 calories*	*15 calories*

WELCH'S FRUIT SNACKS (2¼ OZ BAG)

1 bag	2 bags	1 bag
210 calories	*420 calories*	*210 calories*

REESE'S PEANUT BUTTER CUPS (2¼ OZ PACKET)

3 peanut butter cups (1 packet)	4 peanut butter cups (1⅓ packets)	2 peanut butter cups (⅔ packet)
330 calories	*440 calories*	*220 calories*

SKITTLES ORIGINAL FRUIT (61 G BAG)

1 bag	1⅔ bags	1 bag
250 calories	*410 calories*	*250 calories*

SNICKERS (2.07 OZ BAR)

1 bar	1½ bars	1 bar
280 calories	*420 calories*	*280 calories*

Unless they're made from dried fruit, fruit-flavored snacks contain none of the real thing.

Crackers

12 Triscuit Original
crackers
240

....................+....................

1 bag Kellogg's Low Fat
Granola Crunch Blends
160

....................=....................

400

calories
★ *fiber*

| TYPICAL PORTION | 400-CALORIE PORTION | MEAL PORTION |

GRANOLA BARS, COOKIES, AND PASTRIES

NATURE VALLEY GRANOLA BAR (¾ OZ)

1 bar	4½ bars	1 bar
90 calories	*405 calories*	*90 calories*

KELLOGG'S RICE KRISPIES TREATS (0.78 OZ PIECE)

1 treat	4½ treats	1 treat
90 calories	*405 calories*	*90 calories*

HO HOS (3 OZ PACKAGE)

3 Ho Hos (1 package)	3 Ho Hos (1 package)	1 Ho Ho (⅓ package)
370 calories	*370 calories*	*120 calories*

FAMOUS AMOS CHOCOLATE CHIP COOKIES (3 OZ BAG)

11 cookies (1 bag)	10 cookies (⅞ bag)	5½ cookies (½ bag)
450 calories	*390 calories*	*225 calories*

MINI CHIPS AHOY! (2 OZ BAG)

9 cookies (1 bag)	13 cookies (1½ bags)	9 cookies (1 bag)
270 calories	*405 calories*	*270 calories*

ENTENMANN'S JUMBO ICED HONEY BUN (5.75 OZ)

1 bun	⅔ bun	½ bun
660 calories	*440 calories*	*330 calories*

| TYPICAL PORTION | 400-CALORIE PORTION | MEAL PORTION |

NUTS AND SNACK MIXES

KELLOGG'S LOW FAT GRANOLA CRUNCH BLENDS (1½ OZ BAG)

1 bag	2½ bags	1 bag
160 calories	400 calories	160 calories

TRADITIONAL CHEX MIX (1¾ OZ BAG)

1 bag	1¾ bags	1 bag
220 calories	385 calories	220 calories

PLANTERS TRAIL MIX NUT & CHOCOLATE (2 OZ BAG)

1 bag	1¼ bags	1 bag
320 calories	400 calories	320 calories

PLANTERS SALTED PEANUTS (2 OZ BAG)

1 bag	1¼ bags	1 bag
330 calories	410 calories	330 calories

Trail Mix
1 bag Planters Trail Mix
Nut & Chocolate
_320_

+

1 Kellogg's
Rice Krispies Treat
_90_

=

410
calories
★ _good fats_

Nuts are among the healthiest snacks, with plenty of good fats, fiber, protein, and minerals.

| TYPICAL PORTION | 400-CALORIE PORTION | MEAL PORTION |

GUM AND MINTS

BREATH SAVERS (12-MINT ROLL)

TYPICAL PORTION	400-CALORIE PORTION	MEAL PORTION
12 mints (1 roll)	80 mints (6⅔ rolls)	1 mint (1/12 roll)
60 calories	*400 calories*	*5 calories*

CERTS BREATH MINTS (5-MINT ROLL)

5 mints (1 roll)	80 mints (16 rolls)	1 mint (⅕ roll)
25 calories	*400 calories*	*5 calories*

SUGARLESS GUM (5-STICK PACK)

5 sticks (1 pack)	80 sticks (16 packs)	1 stick (⅕ pack)
25 calories	*400 calories*	*5 calories*

DOUBLEMINT GUM (5-STICK PACK)

5 sticks (1 pack)	40 sticks (8 packs)	1 stick (⅕ pack)
50 calories	*400 calories*	*10 calories*

TIC TAC FRESHMINTS (0.625 OZ BOX)

40 mints (1 box)	200 mints (5 boxes)	5 mints (⅛ box)
80 calories	*400 calories*	*10 calories*

BUBBLE YUM ORIGINAL GUM (5-PIECE PACK)

5 pieces (1 pack)	16 pieces (3⅕ packs)	1 piece (⅕ pack)
125 calories	*400 calories*	*25 calories*

FIXES

1 Watch out for the word *baked*. Per ounce, baked chips have almost as many calories as fried chips. And crackers and cookies, always baked, still contain plenty of fat and calories.

2 Plan to share. Vending machine packs have gotten bigger over the past few years and often are big enough to share with one or two other people. A suitable portion generally is 1 to 2 ounces.

3 Be smart about sodium by choosing snacks that are less salty, like granola bars and cereal bars. Manufacturers are starting to bring down the salt in snack foods, but there's still enough to make you feel parched. Thirst is a particular problem on planes, where the dry air and limited drink service can cause mild dehydration.

4 Go for gum as an almost calorie-free way to burn a few calories chewing, to clean your teeth, and to resist the temptation of the vending machine.

AIRPORT

More choices than ever behind the security gate

Changes in airport and airline security dealt a double whammy to travelers—no more free meals on most flights and much more time to kill in the airport terminal. So use the extra time to your advantage, and pick up food for the plane after you've cleared security. You might even want to burn off a few calories by walking from one end of the terminal to the other to check out your dining options before you buy. Depending on how long you're in the air, you may need to plan ahead for two meals rather than just one.

TYPICAL PORTION	400-CALORIE PORTION	MEAL PORTION

SANDWICHES AND SALADS

QUIZNOS TURKEY CLUB SUB WITH CHEESE AND DRESSING

1 sandwich	½ sandwich	¼ sandwich
815 calories	*410 calories*	*205 calories*

CIBO EXPRESS HARVEST GRILLED VEGGIE WRAP

1 wrap	1 wrap	½ wrap
410 calories	*410 calories*	*205 calories*

MCDONALD'S HONEY MUSTARD SNACK WRAP

1 wrap with crispy chicken	1½ wraps with grilled chicken	1 wrap with grilled chicken
330 calories	*390 calories*	*260 calories*

COBB SALAD WITH LIGHT RANCH DRESSING

1 salad + 4 Tbsp light ranch dressing	1½ salads + 6 Tbsp light ranch dressing	1 salad + 4 Tbsp light ranch dressing
270 calories	*400 calories*	*270 calories*

Cobb Salad

Cobb salad with 4 Tbsp light ranch dressing
270

+

1 glass wine
120

=

390
calories
★ *fruits/veggies*

Flatbread Pizza

2 slices Uno's Roasted Eggplant, Spinach, and Feta Multigrain Thin Crust Pizza
280

························ **+** ························

¾ cup iced café mocha, with fat-free milk
130

························ **=** ························

410

calories

★ *protein*
★ *fiber*

TYPICAL PORTION	400-CALORIE PORTION	MEAL PORTION
UNO'S CHICKEN CAESAR SALAD		
1 salad + 4 Tbsp Caesar dressing	½ salad + 2 Tbsp Caesar dressing	½ salad + 2 Tbsp fat-free vinaigrette
870 calories	*435 calories*	*305 calories*
QUIZNOS RASPBERRY CHIPOTLE CHICKEN SALAD SERVED WITH FLATBREAD (7")		
1 salad + 3 Tbsp cheese + 4 Tbsp raspberry chipotle dressing + flatbread	1 salad + 1 Tbsp cheese + 1 Tbsp raspberry chipotle dressing + ¼ flatbread	½ salad + 1½ Tbsp cheese + 2 Tbsp raspberry chipotle dressing + ½ flatbread
710 calories	*420 calories*	*355 calories*

PIZZAS

UNO'S ROASTED EGGPLANT, SPINACH, AND FETA MULTIGRAIN THIN CRUST PIZZA (10", CUT INTO 6 SLICES)		
6 slices	3 slices	2 slices
840 calories	*420 calories*	*280 calories*
CALIFORNIA PIZZA KITCHEN GOURMET CHEESE PIZZA ON A REGULAR CRUST (9", CUT INTO 6 SLICES)		
6 slices	2½ slices	2 slices
1,000 calories	*420 calories*	*330 calories*

AIRPLANE FOOD

The food served on domestic flights is unpredictable at best. Freebies, if any, on short flights are limited to a very small packet of peanuts or pretzels. You may be served a snack on longer flights, and all airlines offer food to purchase, although much of it is too high in calories for one person. Planning ahead and bringing food is often a better option to the types of choices listed here:

8 oz tomato juice	40 calories
½ oz packet of pretzels	45 calories
½ oz packet of peanuts	80 calories
8 oz orange juice	120 calories
Terra Blues Potato Chips (1 oz)	130 calories
Doritos Munchies Mix (1 oz)	140 calories
Small turkey sandwich with light mayo, baby carrots, fun-size candy	265 calories
Yogurt parfait	310 calories
Ham and cheese croissant with Dijon mayo	340 calories
Cheese and cracker snack tray with nuts, raisins	430 calories
Pringles (4 oz)	480 calories
Mini Oreos (3¾ oz bag)	530 calories
Snack box (combination of chips, nuts, cheese, sausage, dessert, and/or other items)	600–800 calories

Save some calories for a milky coffee drink like a latte or cappuccino. They're great for satisfying hunger and supplying calcium to keep your bones healthy.

Veggie Wrap

½ grilled veggie wrap
205

+

1 medium banana
110

+

½ oz packet of peanuts
80

=

395

calories

★ good fats
★ fiber
★ fruits/veggies

The fat, protein, and fiber combo in peanuts makes them extremely filling and perfect for a long foodless flight.

	TYPICAL PORTION	400-CALORIE PORTION	MEAL PORTION
CALIFORNIA PIZZA KITCHEN GOURMET BUFFALO CHICKEN PIZZA ON A THIN CRUST (9", CUT INTO 6 SLICES)			
	6 slices	2 slices	2 slices
	1,070 calories	360 calories	360 calories

SNACKS

MEDIUM BANANA (7½")			
	1 banana	4 bananas	1 banana
	110 calories	440 calories	110 calories
FLAT PRETZEL CHIPS (6 OZ BAG)			
	66 chips (1 bag)	40 chips (⅗ bag)	11 chips (⅙ bag)
	660 calories	400 calories	110 calories
RAISIN, NUT, AND YOGURT TRAIL MIX (8 OZ BAG)			
	1 bag	⅜ bag	⅛ bag
	1,000 calories	375 calories	125 calories
ROASTED CASHEWS (3.25 OZ BAG)			
	58 cashews (1 bag)	44 cashews (¾ bag)	14 cashews (¼ bag)
	550 calories	420 calories	140 calories

TYPICAL PORTION	400-CALORIE PORTION	MEAL PORTION
SNACK BOX WITH TRAIL MIX, GRANOLA BAR, APPLE SLICES, GRAPES		
1 Tbsp trail mix + 1 granola bar + 2 apple slices + ¼ cup grapes	2⅓ boxes	1 box
170 calories	*400 calories*	*170 calories*
BROWN RICE CRISPS (5 OZ BAG)		
50 crisps (1 bag)	25 crisps (½ bag)	12 crisps (¼ bag)
700 calories	*350 calories*	*175 calories*
SNACK BOX WITH APPLE SLICES, GRAPES, PRETZELS, SWISS CHEESE		
4 apple slices + ¼ cup grapes + 5 pretzel twists + ½ oz Swiss cheese	2 boxes	1 box
195 calories	*390 calories*	*195 calories*
HUMMUS CUP WITH PRETZEL CRISPS (3.5 OZ)		
1 container	1½ containers	1 container
260 calories	*390 calories*	*260 calories*

Frozen Yogurt and Snacks

1 small soft-serve frozen yogurt
240

+

1 snack box with trail mix, granola bar, apple slices, grapes
170

=

410
calories
★ *good fats*

Scone

½ chocolate chip scone
240

+

1 cup fresh fruit
100

+

4 oz orange juice
60

=

400

calories

★ *fruits/veggies*

TYPICAL PORTION	400-CALORIE PORTION	MEAL PORTION

DESSERTS

FRESH FRUIT CUP

1 cup	4 cups	1 cup
100 calories	*400 calories*	*100 calories*

CHOCOLATE CHIP SCONE (4")

1 scone	¾ scone	½ scone
480 calories	*360 calories*	*240 calories*

SOFT-SERVE FROZEN YOGURT

1 large	1 large	1 small
370 calories	*370 calories*	*240 calories*

YOGURT PARFAIT WITH GRANOLA AND BLUEBERRIES (1 CUP)

1 parfait	1 parfait	1 parfait
380 calories	*380 calories*	*380 calories*

BEVERAGES

WINE (5 OZ GLASS)

1 glass	3½ glasses	1 glass
120 calories	*420 calories*	*120 calories*

ICED CAFÉ MOCHA (16 OZ GLASS)

1 glass, made with 2% milk	2 glasses, made with 2% milk	¾ glass, made with fat-fee milk
200 calories	*400 calories*	*130 calories*

FIXES

1 Remember to fill up on water, coffee, tea, and other calorie-free beverages. The air on planes is extremely dry and dehydrating, and you may think that you're hungry when what you need most is something to drink.

2 Pack your meal carefully if you're bringing food from home. Many a traveler has been forced to give up yogurt, salad dressing, even peanut butter and other semisoft or liquid foods to the security screeners.

3 Put in extra effort to choose foods with fresh fruits and vegetables, as well as whole grains. They can be harder to find and harder to eat enough of—4½ cups of fruits and veggies and at least three daily servings of whole grain foods—when you're traveling.

4 Pack your own snacks in right-size portions, and tuck them into your carry-on. Airport mini-marts like Cibo Express offer a lot of options that are the right size and calories for one person.

5 Avoid buying salty snacks like chips that are sold on the plane, unless you're traveling with a friend. The package is too big for just one person, and it's easy to keep on eating.

For better portion control, put sauce or dressing on your sandwich or salad in the terminal rather than during a cramped and bumpy ride.

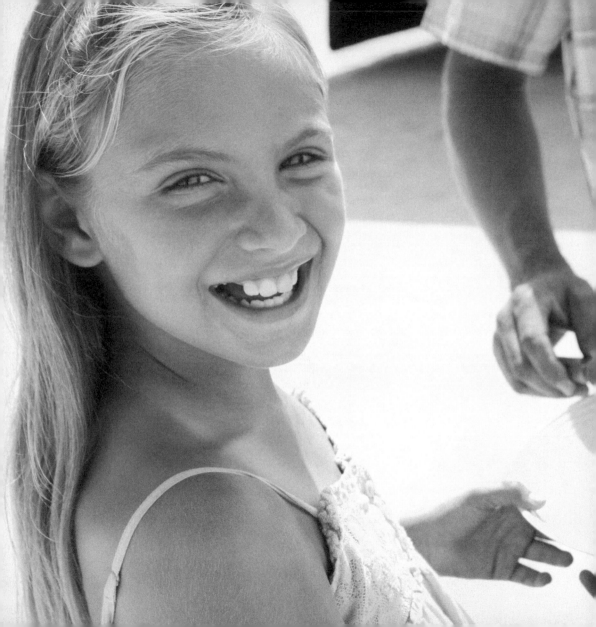

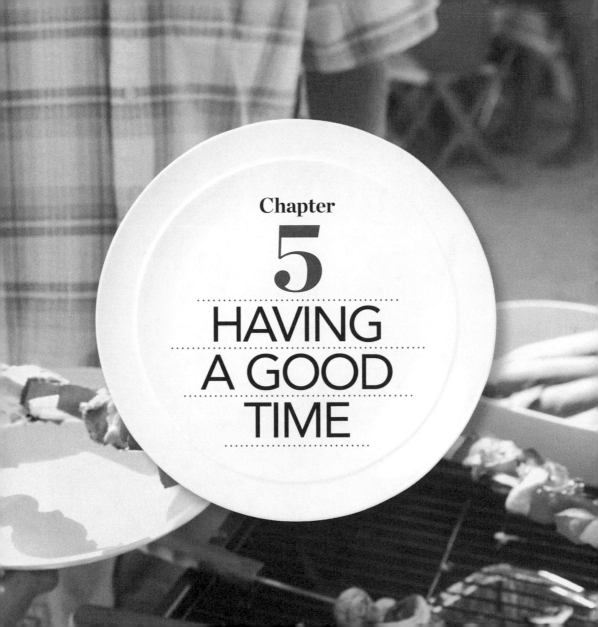

Chapter

5

HAVING
A GOOD
TIME

MOVIES

A favorite spot for candy, popcorn, and soft drinks

It is too bad that snacks you can't see in a dark movie theater still count for calories. And snacks at the theater are really high in price and low in nutrition. To keep temptation under control, make sure that you eat before going to the theater so you can resist the wafting aroma of butter-flavored popcorn, and shop the entire concessions stand before making your pick. Remember that most packages and containers contain at least two 400-calorie portions.

TYPICAL PORTION	400-CALORIE PORTION	MEAL PORTION

CANDY

REESE'S PIECES (4 OZ BOX)

158 pieces (1 box)	105 pieces (⅔ box)	40 pieces (¼ box)
600 calories	*400 calories*	*150 calories*

GOOD & PLENTY (6 OZ BOX)

150 pieces (1 box)	100 pieces (⅔ box)	38 pieces (¼ box)
600 calories	*400 calories*	*150 calories*

WHOPPERS (2¾ OZ BOX)

32 pieces (1 box)	40 pieces (1¼ boxes)	16 pieces (½ box)
320 calories	*400 calories*	*160 calories*

RAISINETS (3½ OZ BOX)

105 pieces (1 box)	105 pieces (1 box)	52 pieces (½ box)
380 calories	*380 calories*	*190 calories*

SOUR PATCH KIDS (3½ OZ BOX)

39 pieces (1 box)	43 pieces (1¹⁄₁₀ boxes)	20 pieces (½ box)
370 calories	*405 calories*	*190 calories*

SKITTLES (7.2 OZ BAG)

200 pieces (1 bag)	100 pieces (½ bag)	50 pieces (¼ bag)
810 calories	*405 calories*	*200 calories*

Candies made with chocolate or nuts are higher in fat than candies that are almost entirely sugar.

Some people find that chewy candies like licorice are more satisfying.

	TYPICAL PORTION	400-CALORIE PORTION	MEAL PORTION
HERSHEY'S SPECIAL DARK CHOCOLATE (6.8 OZ BAR)			
	14 blocks (1 bar) *790 calories*	7 blocks (½ bar) *395 calories*	3½ blocks (¼ bar) *200 calories*
M&MS (5.3 OZ BAG)			
	180 pieces (1 bag) *810 calories*	90 pieces (½ bag) *405 calories*	45 pieces (¼ bag) *200 calories*
DOTS (7½ OZ BOX)			
	68 pieces (1 box) *800 calories*	34 pieces (½ box) *400 calories*	17 pieces (¼ box) *200 calories*
PEANUT M&MS (5.3 OZ BAG)			
	64 pieces (1 bag) *830 calories*	32 pieces (½ bag) *415 calories*	16 pieces (¼ bag) *210 calories*
TWIZZLERS BLACK LICORICE (7 OZ PACKAGE)			
	22 pieces (1 package) *830 calories*	11 pieces (½ package) *415 calories*	5½ pieces (¼ package) *210 calories*
BUTTERFINGER MINIS (3½ OZ BOX)			
	10 bars (1 box) *450 calories*	9 bars (⁹⁄₁₀ box) *405 calories*	5 bars (½ box) *225 calories*

TYPICAL PORTION	400-CALORIE PORTION	MEAL PORTION
REESE'S PEANUT BUTTER CUPS (2¼ OZ PACKAGE)		
4 peanut butter cups (1 package)	3½ peanut butter cups (⅞ package)	2 peanut butter cups (½ package)
440 calories	*385 calories*	*220 calories*
JUNIOR MINTS (4 OZ BOX)		
50 pieces (1 box)	38 pieces (¾ box)	25 pieces (½ box)
540 calories	*410 calories*	*270 calories*

Junior Mints and Reese's Pieces

25 Junior Mints
270

·········· + ··········

40 Reese's Pieces
150

·········· = ··········

420
calories
★ *good fats*

BITE BY
BITE

If you're at a theater that sells loose candy by the pound, use this guide to piece-by-piece calories, and keep total weight at around 3 ounces to stay under 400 calories.

1 Raisinet	3.6 calories
1 Reese's Piece	3.8 calories
1 Good & Plenty	4 calories
1 M&M	4.5 calories
1 Sour Patch Kid	9.5 calories
1 Whopper	10 calories
1 Peanut M&M	13 calories
1 Crunch Dib	13 calories
1 Milk Dud	13 calories
1 Red Twizzler	32.5 calories

Popcorn and Soda

½ small popcorn,
no butter
210

+

16 oz soda
200

=

410
calories

TYPICAL PORTION	400-CALORIE PORTION	MEAL PORTION
MIKE AND IKE (9½ OZ BOX)		
176 pieces (1 box)	66 pieces (⅜ box)	44 pieces (¼ box)
1,070 calories	*400 calories*	*270 calories*
TWIZZLERS RED LICORICE (7 OZ PACKAGE)		
18 pieces (1 package)	12 pieces (⅔ package)	9 pieces (½ package)
590 calories	*390 calories*	*295 calories*
MILK DUDS (5 OZ BOX)		
46 pieces (1 box)	31 pieces (⅔ box)	23 pieces (½ box)
610 calories	*405 calories*	*305 calories*

Popcorn portions vary widely, so look for information on portion size and calories before you buy.

| TYPICAL PORTION | 400-CALORIE PORTION | MEAL PORTION |

OTHER SNACKS

SMALL BUTTERED POPCORN

1 order popcorn (7 cups) + 4 squirts butter (4 Tbsp)	½ order popcorn (3½ cups) + 2 squirts butter (2 Tbsp)	½ order popcorn (3½ cups), no butter
830 calories	*420 calories*	*210 calories*

TORTILLA CHIPS WITH QUESO CHEESE DIP

20 chips + 1 cup dip	10 chips + ½ cup dip	5 chips + ¼ cup dip
920 calories	*460 calories*	*230 calories*

PRETZEL BITES WITH CHEESE DIP

1 order (20 pieces) + ⅓ cup dip	½ order (10 pieces) + 2½ Tbsp dip	½ order (10 pieces), no dip
840 calories	*420 calories*	*300 calories*

HOT DOG ON A BUN (6")

1 hot dog	1¼ hot dogs	1 hot dog
350 calories	*440 calories*	*350 calories*

Hot Dog

1 hot dog
350

+

¼ cup frozen lemonade
75

=

425
calories

Ice Cream and Chocolate

16 Crunch Dibs
200

.... + ...

3½ blocks Hershey's
Special Dark Chocolate
200

.... = ...

400
calories
★ *good fats*

TYPICAL PORTION	400-CALORIE PORTION	MEAL PORTION

ICE CREAM AND BEVERAGES

SODA

32 oz	32 oz	16 oz
400 calories	*400 calories*	*200 calories*

CRUNCH DIBS (9 OZ BOX)

64 pieces (1 box)	32 pieces (½ box)	16 pieces (¼ box)
800 calories	*420 calories*	*200 calories*

SLUSH

32 oz	32 oz	16 oz
440 calories	*440 calories*	*220 calories*

NESTLÉ FROZEN LEMONADE CUP

1 lemonade cup	1⅓ lemonade cups	1 lemonade cup
300 calories	*400 calories*	*300 calories*

HÄAGEN-DAZS VANILLA AND ALMONDS ICE CREAM BAR (3 OZ)

1 bar	1⅓ bars	1 bar
310 calories	*410 calories*	*310 calories*

FIXES

1 Bring an empty plastic sandwich or snack bag to the theater. Count out your 400 Calorie Fix portion, place it in the plastic bag, and then either put away the rest of the bag or share it with someone. Otherwise, you're apt to either lose count of how many pieces you've eaten or continue eating past your limit.

2 Eat candy pieces one at a time and pause for a few minutes between pieces. You will enjoy the flavor more.

3 Drink only water and other calorie-free beverages. Soft drink portions are overly large, and calories from liquids are not as filling as calories from food.

4 Choose the smaller package size over the better deal. It's difficult to know just how much you're eating when sharing a huge bucket of popcorn or tray of nachos. Even smarter: Buy the "kid-size" portion.

Movie theater popcorn is popped in oil, squirted with melted butter, and heavily salted, turning healthy into high calorie.

BALLPARKS, AMUSEMENT PARKS, AND FAIRS

Tastes great, but good nutrition can be a challenge

There's an ever-increasing variety of foods served at stadiums and state fairs across the country and just as many ways to overindulge. Take advantage of mandatory menu labeling in some states to help make your 400-calorie decision easier. Information often isn't available, however, so order small because portion sizes usually run large. Sharing items and taking a bite here and there also can keep you in the calorie ballpark. If you're feeling adventurous, swing by stands with more exotic options to find lower-calorie winners like kebabs.

TYPICAL PORTION	400-CALORIE PORTION	MEAL PORTION

ENTRÉES AND SANDWICHES

RAW OYSTERS WITH COCKTAIL SAUCE

1 dozen oysters + 1 Tbsp cocktail sauce	3 dozen oysters + 3 Tbsp cocktail sauce	1 dozen oysters + 1 Tbsp cocktail sauce
130 calories	*390 calories*	*130 calories*

CHILLED U-PEEL-EM SHRIMP

10 shrimp (½ lb)	25 shrimp (1¼ lb)	10 shrimp (½ lb)
170 calories	*425 calories*	*170 calories*

MEDIUM (6") HOT DOG ON A BUN

1 hot dog	1⅛ hot dogs	½ hot dog
350 calories	*395 calories*	*175 calories*

GRILLED MAHI MAHI SANDWICH ON A KAISER ROLL (3½")

1 Kaiser roll + 3 oz mahi mahi + 1 Tbsp tartar sauce + 2 lettuce leaves + 2 slices tomato	1 sandwich	½ sandwich
360 calories	*360 calories*	*180 calories*

CHICKEN KEBAB (4" with 3 pieces chicken thigh)

1 kebab	2⅓ kebabs	1 kebab
180 calories	*420 calories*	*180 calories*

Hot Dog
½ medium hot dog
175
+
1½ bottles beer
225
=
400
calories

U-Peel-Em Shrimp

10 u-peel-em shrimp
170

.... **+** ....

1 small vanilla
soft-serve cone
230

.... **=** ....

400
calories

★ *protein*

Oysters and Lobster Roll

1 dozen raw oysters +
1 Tbsp cocktail sauce
130

.... **+** ....

½ lobster roll
250

.... **=** ....

380
calories

★ *protein*

TYPICAL PORTION	400-CALORIE PORTION	MEAL PORTION
CHICKEN TENDERS (2") + BARBECUE SAUCE		
4 tenders + 2 Tbsp barbecue sauce	4 tenders + 2 Tbsp barbecue sauce	2 tenders + 1 Tbsp barbecue sauce
400 calories	*400 calories*	*200 calories*
TUNA SALAD SANDWICH ON A KAISER ROLL (3½")		
1 Kaiser roll + ½ cup tuna salad + 2 leaves lettuce + 2 slices tomato	1 sandwich	½ sandwich
430 calories	*430 calories*	*225 calories*
GRILLED SAUSAGE WITH PEPPERS AND ONIONS ON A ROLL (6")		
1 sausage roll	⅞ sausage roll	½ roll
450 calories	*395 calories*	*225 calories*
BEEF KEBAB (4" STRIP SKIRT STEAK)		
2 kebabs	3½ kebabs	2 kebabs
230 calories	*400 calories*	*230 calories*
LOBSTER ROLL ON A BUN		
1 lobster roll	¾ lobster roll	½ lobster roll
500 calories	*375 calories*	*250 calories*
CRAB CAKES		
4 crab cakes	4½ crab cakes	3 crab cakes
370 calories	*420 calories*	*280 calories*

TYPICAL PORTION	400-CALORIE PORTION	MEAL PORTION
FRIED CLAMS		
1 cup clams	⅔ cup clams	½ cup clams
600 calories	*400 calories*	*300 calories*
EMPANADA (3 OZ)		
2 empanadas	1⅓ empanadas	1 empanada
600 calories	*400 calories*	*300 calories*
BABY BACK RIBS		
½ rack (6 ribs)	2½ ribs	2 ribs
930 calories	*390 calories*	*310 calories*

Sausage with Peppers and Onions

½ grilled sausage, peppers, and onions on a roll
225

+

12 fries +
2 Tbsp ketchup
200

=

425
calories

CONDIMENTS

Most condiments add flavor without many calories.

1 tsp mustard	5
2 pickle slices	5
5 Tbsp chopped onions	5
1 Tbsp ketchup	15
½ cup sauerkraut	15
1 Tbsp pickle relish	20
2 Tbsp sautéed onions	60

Pick just one fried food and set your limit at a couple bites, or peel off and toss the fried crust.

TYPICAL PORTION	400-CALORIE PORTION	MEAL PORTION
CORN DOG (6")		
1 corn dog	1 corn dog	1 corn dog
380 calories	*380 calories*	*380 calories*
GRILLED CHICKEN KEBAB SANDWICH		
6½" pita bread + 3 oz grilled chicken thigh + ¼ cup chopped lettuce and tomato + 1 tsp tahini	1 sandwich	1 sandwich
400 calories	*400 calories*	*400 calories*

SNACKS

TYPICAL PORTION	400-CALORIE PORTION	MEAL PORTION
CORN ON THE COB (7" EAR)		
1 ear corn + 2 tsp butter	2⅔ ears corn + 1⅔ Tbsp butter	1 ear corn + 2 tsp butter
150 calories	*380 calories*	*150 calories*
GARLIC BREAD (¾ OZ, 2" PIECE)		
1 piece	2 pieces	1 piece
190 calories	*380 calories*	*190 calories*
FRENCH FRIES		
30 fries + 5 Tbsp ketchup	24 fries + 4 Tbsp ketchup	12 fries + 2 Tbsp ketchup
500 calories	*400 calories*	*200 calories*

TYPICAL PORTION	400-CALORIE PORTION	MEAL PORTION
SMALL BUTTERED POPCORN		
1 order (7 cups) + 4 squirts butter (4 Tbsp)	½ order (3½ cups) + 2 squirts butter (2 Tbsp)	½ order (3½ cups), no butter
830 calories	*420 calories*	*210 calories*
TORTILLA CHIPS WITH QUESO CHEESE DIP		
20 chips + 1 cup dip	10 chips + ½ cup dip	5 chips + ¼ cup dip
920 calories	*460 calories*	*230 calories*

Corn Dog
1 corn dog
·········· **=** ··········
380
calories

FIND THE
FAT

If it's fried, about half its calories or more come from fat:

FOOD	PERCENT CALORIES FROM FAT
French fries	43
Fried Oreo	50
Zeppole	50
Fried clams	53
Chicken tenders	55
Medium onion rings	58

Peanuts

⅓ bag (about 9)
shell-on peanuts
300

··········· + ···········

⅔ glass lemonade
110

··········· = ···········

410

calories

★ *good fats*

	TYPICAL PORTION	400-CALORIE PORTION	MEAL PORTION
MEDIUM ONION RINGS (3")			
	10 onion rings	17 onion rings	10 onion rings
	240 calories	*410 calories*	*240 calories*
LARGE SOFT PRETZEL (5 OZ)			
	1 pretzel	¾ pretzel	½ pretzel
	520 calories	*390 calories*	*260 calories*
SHELL-ON PEANUTS (8 OZ BAG)			
	1 bag (28 shell-on peanuts)	½ bag (14 shell-on peanuts)	⅓ bag (9 shell-on peanuts)
	900 calories	*450 calories*	*300 calories*

SWEETS

DEEP-FRIED OREOS			
	6 Oreos	4 Oreos	1 Oreo
	600 calories	*400 calories*	*100 calories*
COTTON CANDY ON A STICK (4" BALL)			
	2 balls cotton candy	3½ balls cotton candy	1 ball cotton candy
	240 calories	*420 calories*	*120 calories*
BANANA SPLIT DIPPIN' DOTS			
	1 cup Dots	1⅛ cups Dots	½ cup Dots
	340 calories	*380 calories*	*170 calories*

TYPICAL PORTION	400-CALORIE PORTION	MEAL PORTION
CRACKER JACK (2.875 OZ BAG)		
1 bag	1⅛ bags	½ bag
350 calories	395 calories	175 calories
ZEPPOLES WITH POWDERED SUGAR		
3 zeppoles	4 zeppoles	2 zeppoles
300 calories	400 calories	200 calories
MEDIUM CARAMEL APPLE		
1 apple	⅞ apple	½ apple
450 calories	395 calories	225 calories
VANILLA SOFT-SERVE CONE		
1 large cone	1 medium cone + sprinkles	1 small cone
470 calories	400 calories	230 calories
MEDIUM SNOW CONE		
1 cone	1½ cones	1 cone
250 calories	375 calories	250 calories
FUNNEL CAKE (6" CAKE)		
1 cake	1⅓ cakes	1 cake
280 calories	400 calories	280 calories
MEDIUM CANDY APPLE		
1 apple	1⅓ apples	1 apple
300 calories	400 calories	300 calories

Cotton Candy and Funnel Cake

1 ball cotton candy on a stick
120

+

1 funnel cake
280

=

400
calories

Thick Shake

½ container thick or
frozen shake
295

.... + ...

1 zeppole
100

.... = ...

395

calories

All the
calories in
lemonade
come from sugar;
lemon juice
is virtually
calorie free.

BEVERAGES

	TYPICAL PORTION	400-CALORIE PORTION	MEAL PORTION
LIGHT BEER (12 OZ BOTTLE)			
	1 bottle	4 bottles	1 bottle
	100 calories	*400 calories*	*100 calories*
FRESH LEMONADE (12 OZ GLASS)			
	1 glass	2½ glasses	⅔ glass
	160 calories	*400 calories*	*110 calories*
BEER (12 OZ BOTTLE)			
	1 bottle	2⅔ bottles	1 bottle
	150 calories	*400 calories*	*150 calories*
MALTERNATIVE DRINK (16 OZ BOTTLE)			
	1 bottle	1⅓ bottles	¾ bottle
	300 calories	*400 calories*	*230 calories*
THICK OR FROZEN SHAKE (20 OZ GLASS)			
	1 shake	⅔ shake	½ shake
	590 calories	*400 calories*	*295 calories*

FIXES

1 The hot sun can be extremely dehydrating, so be sure to tank up on water, seltzer, and other calorie-free beverages. Avoid spending calories on drinks if you want to keep all 400 meal calories for indulgent foods.

2 Look for foods "on a stick," like grilled chicken kebabs, so you avoid calories from bread. Try corn on the cob as an alternative to a corn dog. Raw shellfish like oysters and shrimp are among the lowest-calorie picks at the beach.

3 Decide before you go: Many ballparks list concession options on their Web sites, and fairs and boardwalks tend to offer the same types of foods. Get as much info ahead of time to find lighter options and regional or nontraditional foods that may be smarter choices.

4 Don't fall for the gimmicky deep-fried pizza, cookies, candy bars, ice cream, and even pickles these days. The calories are not worth it!

5 Portion sizes—and calories—of many foods vary even within the same stadium, fair, or beach, so pick the smallest size order to play it safe.

BARS

Classic drinks and snacks to go with them

Nobody goes into a bar looking for good nutrition, so be sure to collect all your stars in other meals. It's a bonus if you happen to collect a good fats star for eating peanuts or guacamole, or a fruits and veggies star for mixing your drink with orange or tomato juice. Many drinks tend to be large, so plan to share with a friend or ask the bartender for an ultra-small drink in a shot or liqueur glass. Sip and snack slowly to stretch out your calories through the evening.

| TYPICAL PORTION | 400-CALORIE PORTION | MEAL PORTION |

SPIRITS AND MIXED DRINKS

BLOODY MARY (8 OZ GLASS)

1 glass	3½ glasses	1 glass
120 calories	*420 calories*	*120 calories*

COGNAC (2 OZ SNIFTER)

1 snifter	3 snifters	1 snifter
130 calories	*390 calories*	*130 calories*

VODKA (2 OZ SHOT)

1 shot	3 shots	1 shot
130 calories	*390 calories*	*130 calories*

SCOTCH (2 OZ SHOT)

1 shot	3 shots	1 shot
140 calories	*420 calories*	*140 calories*

GIN AND TONIC (8 OZ GLASS)

1 glass	2¾ glasses	1 glass
150 calories	*410 calories*	*150 calories*

RUM AND COKE (8 OZ GLASS)

1 glass	2½ glasses	1 glass
160 calories	*400 calories*	*160 calories*

MARTINI (4 OZ GLASS)

1 glass	1¾ glasses	¾ glass
225 calories	*395 calories*	*170 calories*

Gin and Tonic with Snacks

1 glass gin and tonic
150

+

17 tiny twist pretzels
110

+

¼ cup wasabi peas
120

=

380

calories

Margarita and Chips

½ glass frozen margarita
190

················ **+** ················

10 tortilla chips
145

················ **+** ················

¼ cup guacamole
80

················ **=** ················

415
calories
★ *good fats*

TYPICAL PORTION	400-CALORIE PORTION	MEAL PORTION
SCREWDRIVER (8 OZ GLASS)		
1 glass	2½ glasses	1 glass
170 calories	*425 calories*	*170 calories*
FROZEN MARGARITA (12 OZ GLASS)		
1 glass	1 glass	½ glass
380 calories	*380 calories*	*190 calories*

SPOT THE SUGAR

These mixers are notoriously sweet and high in sugar.

MIXER	SUGAR (G) PER OZ
Rose's Lime	2.1
Orange juice	2.5
Tonic water	2.6
Ginger ale	2.6
Lemon lime soda	2.9
Cola	3.3
Cranberry juice cocktail	3.7
Daiquiri mix	4.5
Sweet and sour mix	5.5
Margarita mix	6.5
Grenadine	18.6

TYPICAL PORTION	400-CALORIE PORTION	MEAL PORTION

COSMO (4 OZ GLASS)

1 glass	2 glasses	1 glass
200 calories	*400 calories*	*200 calories*

FROZEN PIÑA COLADA (12 OZ GLASS)

1 glass	¾ glass	½ glass
500 calories	*375 calories*	*250 calories*

LONG ISLAND ICED TEA (8 OZ GLASS)

1 glass	1 glass	¾ glass
370 calories	*370 calories*	*280 calories*

NONALCOHOLIC

SUGAR-FREE RED BULL (8.4 OZ CAN)

1 can	27 cans	1 can
15 calories	*405 calories*	*15 calories*

GINGER ALE (8 OZ GLASS)

1 glass	5 glasses	1 glass
80 calories	*400 calories*	*80 calories*

RED BULL (8.4 OZ CAN)

1 can	3⅔ cans	1 can
110 calories	*405 calories*	*110 calories*

ORANGE JUICE (8 OZ GLASS)

1 glass	3½ glasses	1 glass
120 calories	*420 calories*	*120 calories*

Buffalo Chicken Wings

1 glass ginger ale
80

+

4 buffalo chicken wings + 2 Tbsp blue cheese dressing
340

=

420
calories

Ask if your Cosmo can be made with light cranberry juice; regular cranberry juice cocktail is much higher in calories.

Beer and Chips

2 bottles light beer
200

.... **+** ....

5 tortilla chips + ¼ cup queso cheese dip
230

.... **=** ....

430

calories

TYPICAL PORTION	400-CALORIE PORTION	MEAL PORTION

BEER AND WINE

LIGHT BEER (12 OZ BOTTLE)

1 bottle	4 bottles	1 bottle
100 calories	*400 calories*	*100 calories*

CHAMPAGNE (5 OZ FLUTE)

1 flute	3½ flutes	1 flute
110 calories	*385 calories*	*110 calories*

WINE (5 OZ GLASS)

1 glass	3½ glasses	1 glass
120 calories	*420 calories*	*120 calories*

BEER (12 OZ BOTTLE)

1 bottle	2⅔ bottles	1 bottle
150 calories	*400 calories*	*150 calories*

PALE ALE (12 OZ BOTTLE)

1 bottle	2 bottles	1 bottle
190 calories	*380 calories*	*190 calories*

STOUT (12 OZ BOTTLE)

1 bottle	2 bottles	1 bottle
200 calories	*400 calories*	*200 calories*

PORTER (12 OZ BOTTLE)

1 bottle	1¾ bottles	1 bottle
220 calories	*385 calories*	*220 calories*

TYPICAL PORTION	400-CALORIE PORTION	MEAL PORTION

SNACKS

GUACAMOLE

1 cup guacamole	1¼ cups guacamole	¼ cup guacamole
320 calories	*400 calories*	*80 calories*

TINY TWIST PRETZELS

34 pretzels	62 pretzels	17 pretzels
220 calories	*400 calories*	*110 calories*

WASABI PEAS

½ cup peas	¾ cup peas	¼ cup peas
240 calories	*360 calories*	*120 calories*

TORTILLA CHIPS

20 chips	28 chips	10 chips
290 calories	*410 calories*	*145 calories*

FRENCH FRIES

12 fries + 2 Tbsp ketchup	24 fries + 4 Tbsp ketchup	12 fries + 2 Tbsp ketchup
200 calories	*400 calories*	*200 calories*

MIXED NUTS

½ cup nuts	½ cup nuts	¼ cup nuts
400 calories	*400 calories*	*200 calories*

Piña Colada and Fries

½ glass frozen piña colada
250

+

9 fries + 1½ Tbsp ketchup
130

=

380
calories

Vodka with Snacks

2 oz shot vodka
130
.... + ...
¼ cup dry roasted
peanuts
210
.... + ...
1 Cheddar bacon
potato skin
70
.... = ...

410

calories

★ *good fats*

TYPICAL PORTION	400-CALORIE PORTION	MEAL PORTION
DRY-ROASTED PEANUTS		
½ cup nuts	½ cup nuts	¼ cup nuts
420 calories	*420 calories*	*210 calories*
CHEDDAR BACON POTATO SKINS		
6 skins	6 skins	3 skins
420 calories	*420 calories*	*210 calories*
CHEESEBURGER SLIDERS		
4 sliders	2 sliders	1 slider
840 calories	*420 calories*	*210 calories*
TORTILLA CHIPS WITH QUESO CHEESE DIP		
20 chips + 1 cup dip	10 chips + ½ cup dip	5 chips + ¼ cup dip
920 calories	*460 calories*	*230 calories*
MEDIUM ONION RINGS (3")		
10 onion rings	17 onion rings	10 onion rings
240 calories	*410 calories*	*240 calories*
BUFFALO CHICKEN WINGS		
8 wings + ¼ cup blue cheese dressing	5 wings + 2½ Tbsp blue cheese dressing	4 wings + 2 Tbsp blue cheese dressing
680 calories	*425 calories*	*340 calories*

FIXES

1 Decide on your drink limit ahead of time, usually a single drink if you want to have a bar snack and still stay within your 400-calorie limit.

2 Order food before you have your first drink. Food in your stomach helps slow absorption of alcohol. And since alcohol lowers inhibitions, you may be more apt to order too much food once you have a drink in your system.

3 Finding healthy bar food is nearly impossible, with a few exceptions like nuts and guacamole. Both have plenty of good fats. But watch the portion since calories add up quickly.

4 Follow every alcohol-containing drink with a calorie-free, nonalcoholic beverage such as water, seltzer, iced tea, or diet cola.

5 Drink as slowly as possible, taking a break between sips, to make your drink last longer. Add ice as needed to keep your drink cold.

6 To cut down on sweetness, ask the bartender to use less of the mixer. Then dilute your drink with seltzer, water, or ice.

All hard liquors, including rum, vodka, gin, whiskey, and brandy, provide 65 to 70 calories per ounce.

PARTIES

Celebrations for adults as well as kids

Let's be realistic—it is hard to stay within your 400-calorie framework at a party, let alone put together a balanced meal. But that doesn't mean that it is impossible. To free up calories, say no to ordinary foods, such as chips and nuts, that you could eat any time. Then decide which foods are really worth the splurge. One of the best strategies is to think small and enjoy your food in one- or two-bite portions, the usual size of "passed" hors d'oeuvres. Pace yourself, especially at parties with separate appetizer, meal, and dessert hours.

HORS D'OEUVRES

TYPICAL PORTION	400-CALORIE PORTION	MEAL PORTION

CRUDITÉS (RAW VEGETABLES)

½ cup	8 cups	½ cup
25 calories	*400 calories*	*25 calories*

SHUMAI (CHINESE SHRIMP DUMPLING)

1 dumpling	16 dumplings	1 dumpling
25 calories	*400 calories*	*25 calories*

MINI CRAB CAKE

1 crab cake	13 crab cakes	1 crab cake
30 calories	*390 calories*	*30 calories*

RAW OYSTERS WITH COCKTAIL SAUCE

3 oysters + 1 tsp cocktail sauce	42 oysters + 5 Tbsp cocktail sauce	3 oysters + 1 tsp cocktail sauce
30 calories	*420 calories*	*30 calories*

PROSCIUTTO

1 slice	13 slices	1 slice
30 calories	*390 calories*	*30 calories*

MINI CHICKEN EGG ROLL

1 egg roll	12 egg rolls	1 egg roll
35 calories	*420 calories*	*35 calories*

CALIFORNIA ROLL

1 piece	10 pieces	1 piece
40 calories	*400 calories*	*40 calories*

Crudités and Dip

1 cup crudités
50

+

5 olives
50

+

2 Tbsp hummus
50

+

6 pita chips
60

+

2 bocconcini and cherry tomato skewers
100

+

2 Tbsp mixed nuts
100

=

410
calories

★ *good fats*
★ *fruits/veggies*

Kids' Birthday Party

10 baby carrots
40

+

½ slice cheese pizza
160

+

½ small cupcake with frosting
120

+

¼ cup vanilla ice cream
70

=

390
calories

TYPICAL PORTION	400-CALORIE PORTION	MEAL PORTION
TUNA ROLL		
1 piece	10 pieces	1 piece
40 calories	*400 calories*	*40 calories*
SPINACH ARTICHOKE DIP		
2 Tbsp dip	1 cup + 2 Tbsp dip	2 Tbsp dip
45 calories	*405 calories*	*45 calories*

KIDS' PARTY

With so many parents onboard the healthy eating bandwagon for kids, you're likely to find at least a few foods to put together for your 400-calorie meal. Remember to save room for dessert!

10 baby carrots	40 calories
10 potato chips	100 calories
1 scoop (½ cup) vanilla ice cream	140 calories
1 cup Chex Mix	190 calories
4 small (⅔ oz) chocolate chip cookies	240 calories
1 slice cheese pizza (14", cut into 8 slices)	320 calories
1 (6") hot dog on a bun	350 calories
Medium (3 oz) yellow cupcake with frosting	530 calories

TYPICAL PORTION	400-CALORIE PORTION	MEAL PORTION
SPICY SALMON ROLL		
1 piece *50 calories*	8 pieces *400 calories*	1 piece *50 calories*
MINI BROCCOLI CHEESE QUICHE		
1 quiche *50 calories*	8 quiches *400 calories*	1 quiche *50 calories*
OLIVES		
5 olives *50 calories*	40 olives *400 calories*	5 olives *50 calories*
PUMPERNICKEL WITH SMOKED SALMON AND EGG		
1 slice pumpernickel snack bread + 2 slices smoked salmon + 1 tsp chopped egg + ½ tsp capers + 1 tsp onion *50 calories*	8 slices *400 calories*	1 slice *50 calories*
HUMMUS		
¼ cup hummus (4 Tbsp) *100 calories*	1 cup hummus *400 calories*	2 Tbsp hummus *50 calories*

Kid-size portions are a great calorie-control tool for adults.

Asian Hors d'Oeuvres

3 shumai
75

.... + ...

3 mini chicken egg rolls
105

.... + ...

4 mini chicken satay skewers
120

.... + ...

3 thin slices flank steak
100

.... = ...

400
calories
★ *protein*

TYPICAL PORTION	400-CALORIE PORTION	MEAL PORTION
SPIRAL HAM		
6 thin slices	40 thin slices	6 thin slices
60 calories	*400 calories*	*60 calories*
MINI CHICKEN SATAY SKEWERS		
2 skewers	13 skewers	2 skewers
60 calories	*390 calories*	*60 calories*
PIGS IN A BLANKET		
1 pig in a blanket	7 pigs in a blanket	1 pig in a blanket
60 calories	*420 calories*	*60 calories*
MINI CORN DOG		
1 corn dog	6½ corn dogs	1 corn dog
60 calories	*390 calories*	*60 calories*
DEVILED EGGS		
1 half egg	7 half eggs	1 half egg
60 calories	*420 calories*	*60 calories*
ROAST BEEF PINWHEEL WRAP		
2 slices	12 slices	2 slices
70 calories	*420 calories*	*70 calories*
TOMATO PROVOLONE PINWHEEL WRAP		
2 slices	12 slices	2 slices
70 calories	*420 calories*	*70 calories*

TYPICAL PORTION	400-CALORIE PORTION	MEAL PORTION
MINI MUSHROOM TURNOVERS		
2 turnovers	10 turnovers	2 turnovers
80 calories	*400 calories*	*80 calories*
SHRIMP COCKTAIL		
3 shrimp + ¼ cup cocktail sauce	12 shrimp + 1 cup cocktail sauce	3 shrimp + ¼ cup cocktail sauce
90 calories	*360 calories*	*90 calories*
ROAST BEEF		
1 thin slice	13 thin slices	3 thin slices
30 calories	*390 calories*	*90 calories*
FLANK STEAK		
3 thin slices	12 thin slices	3 thin slices
100 calories	*400 calories*	*100 calories*
SMALL SPINACH AND CHEESE TARTS		
2 tarts	8 tarts	2 tarts
100 calories	*400 calories*	*100 calories*
SCALLOPS WRAPPED IN BACON		
2 scallops	8 scallops	2 scallops
100 calories	*400 calories*	*100 calories*
MIXED NUTS		
¼ cup nuts	½ cup nuts	2 Tbsp nuts
200 calories	*400 calories*	*100 calories*

Mini Hot Dogs

2 pigs in a blanket + 1 tsp mustard
125

+

1 mini corn dog
60

+

2 halves deviled egg
120

+

1 bottle light beer
100

=

405
calories

Crudités and Cheese

½ cup crudités
25

+

2 mini mushroom
turnovers
80

+

1 oz Brie
90

+

1 oz Cheddar cheese
110

+

6 Ritz crackers
100

=

405
calories

	TYPICAL PORTION	400-CALORIE PORTION	MEAL PORTION
PÂTÉ			
	2 Tbsp pâté	7 Tbsp pâté	2 Tbsp pâté
	120 calories	*420 calories*	*120 calories*
POTATO CHIPS WITH DIP			
	1 oz chips + 2 Tbsp dip	2 oz chips + ¼ cup dip	1 oz chips + 2 Tbsp dip
	200 calories	*400 calories*	*200 calories*
CHEESEBURGER SLIDERS			
	1 slider	2 sliders	1 slider
	210 calories	*420 calories*	*210 calories*

CHEESE

	TYPICAL PORTION	400-CALORIE PORTION	MEAL PORTION
GOAT CHEESE			
	1 oz	5 oz	1 oz
	80 calories	*400 calories*	*80 calories*
BRIE			
	1 oz	4½ oz	1 oz
	90 calories	*405 calories*	*90 calories*
BOCCONCINI AND CHERRY TOMATO MINI-SKEWERS			
	2 skewers	8 skewers	2 skewers
	100 calories	*400 calories*	*100 calories*

TYPICAL PORTION	400-CALORIE PORTION	MEAL PORTION
GOUDA CHEESE		
1 oz	4 oz	1 oz
100 calories	*400 calories*	*100 calories*
CHEDDAR CHEESE		
1 oz	3¾ oz	1 oz
110 calories	*410 calories*	*110 calories*
PARMIGIANO-REGGIANO OR PARMESAN		
1 oz	3½ oz	1 oz
120 calories	*420 calories*	*120 calories*

BREADS AND CRACKERS

TYPICAL PORTION	400-CALORIE PORTION	MEAL PORTION
PITA CHIPS		
3 chips	40 chips	3 chips
30 calories	*400 calories*	*30 calories*
BRUSCHETTA (1½" ROUND + 1 TSP TOPPING)		
1 slice	13 slices	1 slice
30 calories	*390 calories*	*30 calories*
RITZ CRACKERS		
3 crackers	24 crackers	3 crackers
50 calories	*400 calories*	*50 calories*
TRISCUITS		
3 crackers	20 crackers	3 crackers
60 calories	*400 calories*	*60 calories*

Shrimp and Crab Cake

3 shrimp + ¼ cup cocktail sauce
90
+
1 mini crab cake
30
+
4 Tbsp spinach artichoke dip
90
+
3 Triscuits
60
+
1 flute champagne
110
=

380
calories

Salmon and Scallops

1 glass wine
120

·········· **+** ··········

3 slices pumpernickel
with smoked salmon
and egg
150

·········· **+** ··········

2 scallops wrapped
in bacon
100

·········· **+** ··········

6 large strawberries
45

·········· **=** ··········

415

calories

★ *good fats*
★ *fruits/veggies*

TYPICAL PORTION	400-CALORIE PORTION	MEAL PORTION

BEVERAGES

LIGHT BEER (12 OZ BOTTLE)

1 bottle	4 bottles	1 bottle
100 calories	*400 calories*	*100 calories*

CHAMPAGNE (5 OZ FLUTE)

1 flute	3½ flutes	1 flute
110 calories	*385 calories*	*110 calories*

WINE (5 OZ GLASS)

1 glass	3½ glasses	1 glass
120 calories	*420 calories*	*120 calories*

BEER (12 OZ BOTTLE)

1 bottle	2⅔ bottles	1 bottle
150 calories	*400 calories*	*150 calories*

MARTINI (4 OZ GLASS)

1 glass	1¾ glasses	¾ glass
225 calories	*390 calories*	*170 calories*

COSMO (4 OZ GLASS)

1 glass	2 glasses	1 glass
200 calories	*400 calories*	*200 calories*

BITE BY
BITE

Parties are the perfect setting for eating your
400 calories in small bites:

FOOD	CALORIES PER BITE
Cantaloupe ball	5
Pita chip	5
Oyster	10
Spinach artichoke dip	22
Hummus	25
Deviled egg	30
Brownie	30
Mini crab cake	30
Pecan pie	35
Chocolate-covered strawberry	40
Mini mushroom turnover	40
Mini broccoli cheese quiche	40
Brie	45
Scallop wrapped in bacon	50
Chocolate cake	50
Cheddar cheese	55
Paté	60
Strawberry cheesecake	90

Cheeses are around 100 calories per ounce. Hard cheeses like Cheddar and Parmesan are higher in calories than soft cheeses like goat and Brie.

Ditch the crust, and save big on quiches, tarts, and pies.

TYPICAL PORTION	400-CALORIE PORTION	MEAL PORTION

FRUITS AND DESSERTS

CANTALOUPE BALLS

3 balls	120 balls	3 balls
10 calories	400 calories	10 calories

LARGE STRAWBERRIES

2 strawberries	52 strawberries	2 strawberries
15 calories	390 calories	15 calories

BROWNIE (2" SQUARE)

1 brownie	1⅔ brownies	½ brownie
240 calories	400 calories	120 calories

SUGAR COOKIE (1 OZ)

1 cookie	3 cookies	1 cookie
140 calories	420 calories	140 calories

STRAWBERRY CHEESECAKE (1½" SQUARE)

1 square	2¼ squares	1 square
180 calories	405 calories	180 calories

CHOCOLATE CAKE WITH CHOCOLATE FROSTING (4 OZ SLICE)

1 slice	1 slice	½ slice
410 calories	410 calories	205 calories

PECAN PIE (8", CUT INTO 6 SLICES)

1 slice	⅔ slice	½ slice
570 calories	380 calories	285 calories

FIXES

1 Consider doubling up by combining two meals for a total of 800 calories. Parties are special occasions that should be enjoyed . . . within reason!

2 Always eat before you drink. Alcohol hits harder on an empty stomach and also may loosen your inhibitions enough to undo your best intentions. And stick to one alcoholic drink max, saving the rest of your calories for food.

3 Hold an alcohol-free drink—preferably a calorie-free one, such as sparkling water—in one hand so that it's harder to eat.

4 Avoid standing next to snacks in bowls, and stand as far away from the bar and food tables as possible to lessen temptation. Better yet, use party time to socialize or even to burn calories dancing or taking part in kids' games.

5 Seek out raw veggies and fresh fruit for a low-calorie way to fill your plate. And dip with vegetables rather than with bread or chips.

6 The raw seafood bar and the sashimi platter are filled with low-calorie raw fish options. Choose cocktail sauce rather than higher-calorie tartar sauce, and go easy on sushi—the rice adds calories.

BANQUETS AND WEDDINGS

Best picks for sit-down celebrations

You're usually locked into a set menu at a sit-down banquet or wedding without many options for changing what's on your plate. If printed menus are on the table, you have the opportunity to plan your meal ahead of time. You may even decide to skip a course or two to keep calories under control.

Plain grilled fish, seafood, and chicken often are calorie-smart bets when available, and a vegetarian plate may be a lighter meal. Portions generally are on the large side, so don't hesitate to leave food on your plate or request smaller portions if food is dished out at the table.

| TYPICAL PORTION | 400-CALORIE PORTION | MEAL PORTION |

APPETIZERS

SHRIMP COCKTAIL

3 shrimp + ¼ cup cocktail sauce	12 shrimp + 1 cup cocktail sauce	3 shrimp + ¼ cup cocktail sauce
90 calories	*360 calories*	*90 calories*

MIXED GREEN SALAD with lettuce, dried cranberries, pecans, blue cheese, balsamic vinaigrette dressing

1 cup lettuce + 1 Tbsp each dried cranberries, pecans, blue cheese + 1 Tbsp balsamic vinaigrette dressing	2 salads	½ salad
200 calories	*400 calories*	*100 calories*

FRESH FRUIT SALAD

1 cup	4 cups	1 cup
100 calories	*400 calories*	*100 calories*

Salad

1 mixed green salad with lettuce, dried cranberries, pecans, blue cheese, balsamic vinaigrette dressing
200

+

½ slice carrot cake
225

=

425
calories

★ *good fats*
★ *fruits/veggies*

Chicken Breast

1 cup fresh fruit salad
100

+

½ cup rice pilaf
140

+

3 oz roast
chicken breast
140

=

380

calories

★ *protein*
★ *fruits/veggies*

TYPICAL PORTION	400-CALORIE PORTION	MEAL PORTION

BREADS AND ROLLS

ITALIAN BREAD (2" SLICE) + BUTTER

1 slice + 2 pats butter	2 slices + 3 pats butter	½ slice + 1 pat butter
210 calories	*390 calories*	*105 calories*

SMALL DINNER ROLL (2") + BUTTER

2 rolls + 2 pats butter	3½ rolls + 3½ pats butter	1 roll + 1 pat butter
220 calories	*390 calories*	*110 calories*

FIND THE
FAT

These words usually are a dead giveaway for fat and calories:

- Au gratin
- Au poivre
- Bisque
- Creamed
- Crisp
- Croquette
- En croûte
- Fried
- Parmesan
- Sauce
- Scalloped

TYPICAL PORTION	400-CALORIE PORTION	MEAL PORTION

ENTRÉES

CHICKEN PICCATA WITH PEPPERS

6 oz	9 oz	3 oz
260 calories	*390 calories*	*130 calories*

ROAST CHICKEN BREAST

6 oz	9 oz	3 oz
280 calories	*420 calories*	*140 calories*

CHICKEN AND SPANISH RICE WITH CHEESE SAUCE

1½ cups	1⅓ cups	½ cup
450 calories	*400 calories*	*150 calories*

FLANK STEAK WITH TERIYAKI SAUCE

6 oz	7 oz	3 oz
360 calories	*420 calories*	*180 calories*

GRILLED SALMON

6 oz	6⅔ oz	3 oz
360 calories	*400 calories*	*180 calories*

FRIED CHICKEN DRUMSTICK

2 drumsticks	2 drumsticks	1 drumstick
380 calories	*380 calories*	*190 calories*

ROAST BEEF (1 OZ SLICE)

6 slices	6 slices	3 slices
380 calories	*380 calories*	*190 calories*

Roast Beef

3 shrimp with ¼ cup cocktail sauce
90
+
3 slices roast beef
190
+
½ cup broccoli au gratin
100
=

380
calories
★ *protein*

Most cuts of salmon and beef of the same sizes have about the same number of calories.

Baked Ziti

½ slice Italian bread +
1 pat butter
105

·········· **+** ··········

½ cup baked ziti
210

·········· **+** ··········

1 cup sautéed broccoli
90

·········· **=** ··········

405
calories

★ *fruits/veggies*

	TYPICAL PORTION	400-CALORIE PORTION	MEAL PORTION
FILET MIGNON			
	8 oz	6⅓ oz	3 oz
	500 calories	*400 calories*	*190 calories*
BAKED ZITI			
	1 cup	1 cup	½ cup
	420 calories	*420 calories*	*210 calories*
ROAST HAM (2 OZ SLICE)			
	3 slices	3 slices	1½ slices
	420 calories	*420 calories*	*210 calories*
MEAT LOAF (1", 3 OZ SLICE)			
	1 slice	1 slice	½ slice
	430 calories	*430 calories*	*215 calories*

Banquet vegetables usually are higher in calories because they're made with extra oil and butter.

TYPICAL PORTION	400-CALORIE PORTION	MEAL PORTION
FRIED CHICKEN BREAST		
8 oz	5 oz	3 oz
580 calories	*360 calories*	*220 calories*
BAKED HADDOCK WITH LEMON-BUTTER SAUCE		
6 oz haddock + 1½ Tbsp lemon-butter sauce	7 oz haddock + 1⅔ Tbsp lemon-butter sauce	4 oz haddock + 1 Tbsp lemon-butter sauce
350 calories	*400 calories*	*230 calories*

SIDE DISHES

GLAZED CARROTS		
1 cup	5 cups	½ cup
80 calories	*400 calories*	*40 calories*
SAUTÉED GREEN BEANS AMANDINE		
1 cup	2½ cups	½ cup
160 calories	*400 calories*	*80 calories*
SAUTÉED BROCCOLI		
1 cup	4½ cups	1 cup
90 calories	*405 calories*	*90 calories*
ROASTED POTATOES		
1 cup	2¼ cups	½ cup
180 calories	*405 calories*	*90 calories*

Haddock

½ mixed green salad with lettuce, dried cranberries, pecans, blue cheese, balsamic vinaigrette dressing
100
+
4 oz baked haddock + 1 Tbsp lemon-butter sauce
230
+
1 cup sautéed broccoli
90
=

420
calories

★ *protein*
★ *good fats*
★ *fruits/veggies*

Flank Steak

1 small dinner roll +
1 pat butter
110

···················· **+** ····················

½ cup broccoli au gratin
100

···················· **+** ····················

3 oz flank steak with
teriyaki sauce
180

···················· **=** ····················

390
calories
★ *protein*

TYPICAL PORTION	400-CALORIE PORTION	MEAL PORTION
MASHED POTATOES		
1 cup mashed potatoes + 1 pat butter	2 cups mashed potatoes + 2 pats butter	½ cup mashed potatoes, no butter
210 calories	*420 calories*	*90 calories*
BROCCOLI AU GRATIN		
1 cup	2 cups	½ cup
200 calories	*400 calories*	*100 calories*
RICE PILAF		
1 cup	1½ cups	½ cup
280 calories	*420 calories*	*140 calories*
CREAMED SPINACH		
1 cup	1¼ cups	½ cup
320 calories	*400 calories*	*160 calories*
POTATOES AU GRATIN		
1 cup	1¼ cups	½ cup
320 calories	*400 calories*	*160 calories*
MACARONI AND CHEESE		
1 cup	1 cup	½ cup
360 calories	*360 calories*	*180 calories*

TYPICAL PORTION	400-CALORIE PORTION	MEAL PORTION

DESSERTS

SLICED STRAWBERRIES

1 cup	8 cups	1 cup
50 calories	*400 calories*	*50 calories*

WHIPPED CREAM

¼ cup	1 cup	2 Tbsp
100 calories	*400 calories*	*50 calories*

LARGE CHOCOLATE-COVERED STRAWBERRY

1 strawberry	5 strawberries	1 strawberry
80 calories	*400 calories*	*80 calories*

WEDDING CAKE (4 OZ SLICE)

1 slice	1 slice	½ slice
400 calories	*400 calories*	*200 calories*

CHOCOLATE CAKE WITH CHOCOLATE FROSTING (4 OZ SLICE)

1 slice	1 slice	½ slice
410 calories	*410 calories*	*205 calories*

CARROT CAKE (4 OZ SLICE)

1 slice	1 slice	½ slice
450 calories	*450 calories*	*225 calories*

Salmon

3 oz grilled salmon
180

+

½ cup
potatoes au gratin
160

+

1 cup
sliced strawberries
50

=

390

calories

★ *protein*
★ *good fats*
★ *fruits/veggies*

Cake and Champagne

1 flute champagne
110

········· **+** ·········

½ slice wedding cake
200

········· **+** ·········

1 large chocolate-covered strawberry
80

········· **=** ·········

390
calories
★ *good fats*

TYPICAL PORTION	400-CALORIE PORTION	MEAL PORTION

BEVERAGES

CHAMPAGNE (5 OZ FLUTE)

1 flute	3½ flutes	1 flute
110 calories	*385 calories*	*110 calories*

WINE (5 OZ GLASS)

1 glass	3½ glasses	1 glass
120 calories	*420 calories*	*120 calories*

Dilute your drink with water, seltzer, or club soda to stretch out the calories.

FIXES

1 Avoid the most obvious calorie trap by asking for salad dressing on the side and then using just a drizzle. Or request oil and vinegar on the side.

2 Try to scrape off as much sauce as possible, and skip buttery sauces altogether. A tablespoon of butter sauce can dish up close to 100 calories.

3 Skip breaded coatings like the crust on fried chicken or cutlets.

4 Choose just one starch, either bread or potato or rice, and keep your portion at around one tennis ball, usually about 100 calories.

5 Leave half your food on your plate.

6 Save room for cake by eating small portions of just one or two other foods. Then share a slice of cake to keep your dessert at around 200 calories.

Roast Ham

1½ slices roast ham
210

+

½ cup glazed carrots
40

+

½ cup
potatoes au gratin
160

=

410

calories

★ *protein*
★ *fruits/veggies*

COOKOUTS

Classics from the grill plus favorite sides and salads

Who doesn't love a cookout or BBQ? You usually have plenty to choose from—chips and other snacks, fresh vegetables, an assortment of grilled dishes, several side salads, and both fruit and baked goods for dessert. And count on lemonade, iced tea, beer, and wine to drink. Plan your plate carefully from the various available options so that you can keep within your 400-calorie framework. It can be hard to limit yourself to just a couple of foods, so take just small portions of your higher-calorie favorites . . . and enjoy every bite.

TYPICAL PORTION	400-CALORIE PORTION	MEAL PORTION

APPETIZERS

CRUDITÉS (RAW VEGETABLES)

1 cup	8 cups	1 cup
50 calories	*400 calories*	*50 calories*

POTATO CHIPS

20 chips	40 chips	5 chips
200 calories	*400 calories*	*50 calories*

ONION DIP

½ cup	1 cup	¼ cup (4 Tbsp)
200 calories	*400 calories*	*100 calories*

TORTILLA CHIPS WITH SALSA

18 chips + ¼ cup salsa	27 chips + ⅓ cup salsa	9 chips + 2 Tbsp salsa
280 calories	*420 calories*	*140 calories*

ENTRÉES

CHILI CON CARNE WITH BEANS

1 cup	1⅓ cups	¼ cup
300 calories	*400 calories*	*75 calories*

CHICKEN DRUMSTICK

2 drumsticks	3⅔ drumsticks	1 drumstick
220 calories	*405 calories*	*110 calories*

Chicken Drumsticks

9 tortilla chips + 2 Tbsp salsa
140

+

2 chicken drumsticks
220

+

5 grilled asparagus spears
35

=

395
calories

★ *protein*
★ *fruits/veggies*

Veggie Burger

1 cup crudités
50

.... **+** ....

Veggie burger
on a bun with
1 lettuce leaf,
1 slice tomato,
1 Tbsp ketchup
245

.... **+** ....

2 chocolate chip
cookies
120

.... **=** ....

415

calories
★ *fruits/veggies*

TYPICAL PORTION	400-CALORIE PORTION	MEAL PORTION
BEEF KEBAB WITH VEGETABLES (6" with 3 pieces meat and 3 pieces vegetables)		
3 kebabs	2⅔ kebabs	1 kebab
450 calories	*400 calories*	*150 calories*
BABY BACK RIBS		
4 ribs	2¾ ribs	1 rib
620 calories	*410 calories*	*155 calories*
MEATLESS HOT DOG (1½ OZ) ON A BUN		
1 hot dog + 1 bun	2½ hot dogs + 2½ buns	1 hot dog + 1 bun
165 calories	*410 calories*	*165 calories*
BRISKET		
6 oz	7 oz	3 oz
340 calories	*400 calories*	*170 calories*
FLANK STEAK		
6 oz	7 oz	3 oz
360 calories	*420 calories*	*180 calories*
VEGGIE BURGER (2½ OZ) ON A BUN		
1 patty + 1 bun	1¾ patties + 1¾ buns	1 patty + 1 bun
220 calories	*385 calories*	*220 calories*

CONDIMENTS

A plain burger or dog can be pretty boring, especially lower-fat varieties, so add flavor and satisfaction with one or more condiments.

2 dill pickle slices	0 calories
1 lettuce leaf	5 calories
1 tomato slice	5 calories
1 Tbsp chopped onions	5 calories
1 tsp mustard	5 calories
1 pickle spear	5 calories
2 Tbsp roasted red peppers	10 calories
1 Tbsp ketchup	15 calories
2 sweet pickle slices	15 calories
1 Tbsp pickle relish	20 calories
1 Tbsp blue cheese	30 calories
1 slice bacon	40 calories
2 Tbsp barbecue sauce	50 calories
2 Tbsp sautéed mushrooms	55 calories
¼ cup sliced avocado	60 calories
2 Tbsp sautéed onions	60 calories
1 slice American cheese	70 calories

Eat your burger topless, and save 60 calories. Switch from beef to a veggie burger, and save another 130 calories.

Lean Burger

1 lean beef burger
on a bun with 1 lettuce
leaf, 1 tomato slice,
1 Tbsp ketchup
330

·········· **+** ··········

¼ cup sliced avocado
60

·········· **=** ··········

390
calories

★ protein
★ good fats

TYPICAL PORTION	400-CALORIE PORTION	MEAL PORTION
TURKEY DOG (1¾ OZ) ON A BUN		
1 hot dog + 1 bun	1¾ hot dogs + 1¾ buns	1 hot dog + 1 bun
220 calories	*385 calories*	*220 calories*
HOT ITALIAN SAUSAGE		
6 oz	5 oz	3 oz
460 calories	*380 calories*	*230 calories*
BARBECUE CHICKEN		
2 thighs + 2 Tbsp sauce	3 thighs + 3 Tbsp sauce	2 thighs + 2 Tbsp sauce
270 calories	*405 calories*	*270 calories*
BEEF HOT DOG (1¾ OZ) ON A BUN		
1 hot dog + 1 bun	1½ hot dogs + 1½ buns	1 hot dog + 1 bun
270 calories	*405 calories*	*270 calories*
BISON BURGER (3 OZ PATTY) ON A BUN		
2 patties + 2 buns	1½ patties + 1½ buns	1 patty + 1 bun
540 calories	*405 calories*	*270 calories*
LEAN BEEF (10% FAT) BURGER (3 OZ PATTY) ON A BUN		
2 patties + 2 buns	1⅓ patties +1⅓ buns	1 patty + 1 bun
610 calories	*415 calories*	*305 calories*

TYPICAL PORTION	400-CALORIE PORTION	MEAL PORTION
TURKEY BURGER (3 OZ PATTY) ON A BUN		
2 patties + 2 buns	1⅓ patties + 1⅓ buns	1 patty + 1 bun
620 calories	*420 calories*	*310 calories*
BEEF (20% FAT) BURGER (3 OZ PATTY) ON A BUN		
2 patties + 2 buns	1⅛ patties + 1⅛ buns	1 patty + 1 bun
700 calories	*395 calories*	*350 calories*

BUNS

An ordinary bun is your best bet for calorie control. Fancier options like hard rolls and brioche can take up at least half your meal calories.

Light bun	80
Whole wheat bun	110
Regular hamburger or hot dog bun	120
Hard roll	170
Brioche	240

Italian Sausage

¼ cup potato salad
80

·················· **+** ··················

¼ cup cole slaw
90

·················· **+** ··················

3 oz hot Italian sausage
230

·················· **=** ··················

400
calories

TYPICAL PORTION	400-CALORIE PORTION	MEAL PORTION

SALADS AND SIDE DISHES

GRILLED ASPARAGUS

5 spears	60 spears	5 spears
35 calories	*420 calories*	*35 calories*

POTATO SALAD

1 cup	1¼ cups	¼ cup
320 calories	*400 calories*	*80 calories*

SMALL DINNER ROLL (2")

1 roll	5 rolls	1 roll
80 calories	*400 calories*	*80 calories*

COLE SLAW

1 cup	1 cup	¼ cup
360 calories	*360 calories*	*90 calories*

GRILLED VEGETABLES

1 slice eggplant + ½ red pepper + ½ portobello cap	4½ slices eggplant + 2¼ red peppers + 2¼ portobello caps	1 slice eggplant + ½ red pepper + ½ portobello cap
90 calories	*405 calories*	*90 calories*

MACARONI SALAD

1 cup	⅞ cup	¼ cup
440 calories	*385 calories*	*110 calories*

TYPICAL PORTION	400-CALORIE PORTION	MEAL PORTION
GRILLED VEGETABLES MARINATED IN VINAIGRETTE		
1 cup	3⅔ cups	1 cup
110 calories	*405 calories*	*110 calories*
VEGETARIAN BAKED BEANS		
1 cup	1⅔ cups	½ cup
240 calories	*400 calories*	*120 calories*
CORN ON THE COB (7" EAR)		
1 ear corn + 2 pats butter	2⅔ ears corn + 1⅔ Tbsp butter	1 ear corn + 2 pats butter
150 calories	*380 calories*	*150 calories*
MACARONI AND CHEESE		
1 cup	1⅛ cups	½ cup
360 calories	*405 calories*	*180 calories*
GARLIC BREAD (2" SLICE)		
1 slice	2 slices	1 slice
190 calories	*380 calories*	*190 calories*

Grilled Salmon

3 oz grilled salmon
180

+

1 cup grilled vegetables marinated in vinaigrette
110

+

⅔ glass lemonade
110

=

400
calories

★ *protein*
★ *good fats*
★ *fruits/veggies*

Beef Kebab

1 beef kebab with
vegetables
150

························ **+** ························

1 ear corn on the cob +
2 pats butter
150

························ **+** ························

1 wedge watermelon
90

························ **=** ························

390
calories

★ *fruits/veggies*

TYPICAL PORTION	400-CALORIE PORTION	MEAL PORTION

FRUIT AND DESSERTS

WATERMELON (1" WEDGE)

1 wedge	4 wedges	1 wedge
90 calories	*360 calories*	*90 calories*

FRUIT SALAD

1 cup	4 cups	1 cup
100 calories	*400 calories*	*100 calories*

CHOCOLATE CHIP COOKIES (⅔ OZ EACH)

3 cookies	6⅔ cookies	2 cookies
180 calories	*400 calories*	*120 calories*

SPOT THE
SUGAR

Many favorite barbecue sauces and condiments
get most of their calories from added sugar:

- Ketchup
- Barbecue sauce
- Steak sauce
- Pickle relish
- Sweet pickles
- Mango salsa
- Sauce on baked beans

TYPICAL PORTION	400-CALORIE PORTION	MEAL PORTION
PEANUT BUTTER COOKIES (⅔ OZ EACH)		
3 cookies	6⅔ cookies	2 cookies
180 calories	*400 calories*	*120 calories*
ICE CREAM		
½ cup	1½ cups	½ cup
140 calories	*420 calories*	*140 calories*
S'MORES		
2 s'mores	2 s'mores	1 s'more
320 calories	*320 calories*	*160 calories*
BROWNIE (2" SQUARE)		
1 brownie	1⅔ brownies	1 brownie
240 calories	*400 calories*	*240 calories*

Meatless Hot Dog

5 potato chips
50

+

1 Tbsp onion dip
25

+

Meatless hot dog
on a bun
165

+

1 s'more
160

=

400
calories

Instead
of a s'more,
toast a couple of
marshmallows
at 25 calories
apiece.

Baby Back Rib

1 cup crudités +
¼ cup onion dip
150

·········· + ··········

1 baby back rib
155

·········· + ··········

1 bottle light beer
100

·········· = ··········

405
calories
★ *fruits/veggies*

TYPICAL PORTION	400-CALORIE PORTION	MEAL PORTION

BEVERAGES

SWEET ICED TEA (12 OZ GLASS)

1 glass	3½ glasses	⅔ glass
120 calories	*420 calories*	*80 calories*

SANGRIA (12 OZ GLASS)

1 glass	1½ glasses	⅓ glass
270 calories	*405 calories*	*90 calories*

LIGHT BEER (12 OZ BOTTLE)

1 bottle	4 bottles	1 bottle
100 calories	*400 calories*	*100 calories*

LEMONADE (12 OZ GLASS)

1 glass	2½ glasses	⅔ glass
160 calories	*400 calories*	*110 calories*

WINE (5 OZ GLASS)

1 glass	3½ glasses	1 glass
120 calories	*420 calories*	*120 calories*

BEER (12 OZ BOTTLE)

1 bottle	2⅔ bottles	1 bottle
150 calories	*400 calories*	*150 calories*

FIXES

1 Limit yourself to one main dish item, for example, a hamburger or a hot dog, and build your meal from there. Unless you go meatless, doubling up on burgers or dogs will put you over 400 calories.

2 Load up your plate with raw veggies and salad greens since they're virtually calorie free. If you have a choice of dressing, go for one that is lower in calories.

3 Veggie salads may look deceptively healthy, but if they look creamy or glisten and have oil slicks, they're likely to be full of fat and calories.

4 Seek out fruit—watermelon is one of the lowest-calorie melons, and fruit salad tops out at about 100 calories per cup.

5 Enjoy activities that take you away from the food tables, like Frisbee, swimming, or playing ball.

INDEX

The EAT Anything, *Anywhere* PLAN!

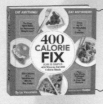

400 Calorie Fix lets you eat anywhere—restaurants, ballparks, even parties!—and still fix your weight loss problems forever. Lose up to 11 pounds in just 2 weeks with the world's easiest weight loss plan.

400 Calorie Fix Tracker
Get the most from **400 Calorie Fix** with this inspirational food and activity journal!

400 Calorie Fix Workout
A metabolism-boosting cardio and strength routine proven to burn 400 calories with each workout.

400 Calorie Fix Cookbook
For the food lover in you, this beautiful volume features 400 all-new 400-calorie meals to cook at home.

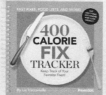

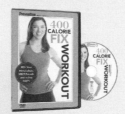

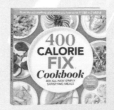

Visit 400CalorieFix.com and order your copies today.